Insight into Piece

Synopsis

Crafted by the author (not a ghost writer), *Insight into Piece* by Kevin Raftery is an interesting and original, sharp-witted book of articles (with a few unusual short-stories thrown in for good measure) featuring multiple styles and genres comprising local, national and even international themes. The pieces appeal to all age groups and range from the insightful, the psychological, the political, the factual and the social.

Written over a seven-year period (2011-2018) barring one or two exceptions, Kevin expertly focuses the critical spotlight on the institutions that govern us, simultaneously recording important socio-historical facts of the time, sometimes controversially. All the events catalogued can be cross-referenced with current affairs of today to proffer an entertaining twist to reading proceedings. These real-life events include the fascinating fly on wall *Inside O' Connor* series which documents real life in rehab for those predisposed to addiction problems.

Covering topics including human nature, travel, disability, addiction and mental health, Insight into Piece contains over 140 articles each written in Kevin's 'unheard' but distinct narrative voice.

Insight into Piece

KEVIN RAFTERY

Matador
9 Priory Business Park,
Wistow Road, Kibworth Beauchamp,
Leicestershire. LE8 0RX
Tel: 0116 279 2299
Email: books@troubador.co.uk
Web: www.troubador.co.uk/matador
Twitter: @matadorbooks

ISBN 978 1789016 291

British Library Cataloguing in Publication Data.
A catalogue record for this book is available from the British Library.

Printed and bound in Great Britain by 4edge Limited
Typeset in 11pt Minion Pro by Troubador Publishing Ltd, Leicester, UK

Matador is an imprint of Troubador Publishing Ltd

Remembering those deceased family members who
were interested in my welfare – it was a long time coming

With thanks to the stranger at the Gladstone Pottery Museum, who, on hearing me relay my full name over the telephone said:

"Kevin Raftery? You write some good stuff."

The Self-belief system is a fragile, precariously shifting phenomenon.

Contents

Insight Definition:

Insight is a precise and perceptive observation of what lies behind the veneer, enabling the re-examination of prevailing convention.

Business as Usual for the Haves and the Have-nots

The popular TV show *Dragon's Den* is a farce. The most essential juncture in the business cycle for entrepreneurs is securing orders for their product or service and/or sourcing stockists or customers in order to sell that product. Instead, 'contestants' on *Dragon's Den* are, by and large, already established and have accrued some sort of profit and customer base, but are pitching to venture capitalists to expand their respective businesses.

But what about the start-up impresarios who have no capital at all?

There are few organisations around to assist those without any resources or collateral. Free seminars and suchlike can be accessed (which can also see local businesses peddling their wares) although online facilities like crowdfunding are not to everyone's liking. When applying to funding organisations online, one's application can be rejected for a whole array of reasons. Investors, or those lauding over funds, are mostly looking for hi-tech companies to invest in to meet their tick-box prerequisites.

Grants (or at least loans) should be made available to assist with fees that are amassed at this important crossroads in the corporate cycle (after finalising the business plan). This would include equipment, accountant's charges, trademarks, start-up advertising, websites, and perhaps the most important of all, representatives or agents to help with accessing contacts who may be in the position to sell the product/service.

In 2015, European monies managed by local authorities/agencies came with the requirement that, if you wanted to apply to the Specialist Intensive Assistance Fund (for example), you could claim £4,500 for specialist external consultancy advice, only on condition that the one applying to the fund spent £18,000 themselves.

When this anomaly was challenged, in that ordinary people have not got £18,000, one 'professional' responded that they should not be going into business then (or words to that effect).

Then we have the chamber of commerce, the answer to the business novice's prayer. There seem to be workshops available from time to time, but real help is non-existent. Recently, chambers were undertaking their quarterly economic survey. Would you believe that data from this is used by the Bank of England's monetary policy committee, as one of its key benchmarks when setting interest rates? HM Treasury and the independent Office for Budget Responsibility also use the data to put together their forecasts for the UK's economic performance.

Economic doom and gloom is forecast, I am afraid, if the lack of initiatives for new business start-up assistance is factored into the statistics.

In the real world, individuals from an ordinary background who manage to establish a company when they have no contacts, capital or collateral (some don't even have an income) are a paucity.

During a chambers workshop, I came across one hard-working young man attempting to set up his own company but had no capital at all. He ended up running around in circles. Most importantly, a vehicle (van) was required so that the business could be run efficiently. A loan of a vehicle until the business is up and running could be one way forward to allow those in the 'non-capital' bracket to institute their concern/s. Then, of course, when that business becomes successful it will be contributing to a strong local/national/international economy and employing people too.

The have-nots in the business community will no doubt question whether their lack of progression in business circles is down to issues around social mobility. Everybody has a right to assert their business acumen, without the disadvantage of financial constraints due to social origin.

Our 'fair and democratic' system seems to afford those with vast amounts of wealth to accumulate even more, while others cannot even get on the ladder. It's not what you know, it's who you know.

Take media construct Victoria Beckham, whose job description in 2017 states that she is a singer (don't snigger), actress (?) and philanthropist (a philanthropist supposedly promotes the welfare of others, especially with generous donations to good causes). Ms Beckham is now worth $450 million. Note dollars and not pounds.

Perhaps *Dragon's Den* should go one step further and introduce the celebrity version of the show to enable the mega-rich to become even richer. Yes, our own Vicky Adams could enter the Den, flogging her Golden Balls range. Now let's see: forget the signature gowns, they're so last winter. The elegant, fluid halterneck dress (with open back) cut from Bordeaux silk layered with georgette, featuring multicoloured abstract print (as seen on the Victoria Beckham website in 2017) is a snip at £2,275, and it's gross to boot. Not to mention those flat, pointy slippers in glossy black calf leather (poor little cow) with twin studded buckles, to guard against that dusty Den floor. If Victoria really wanted to make an impression with the even wealthier Dragons, who would have the power to enable her to become as well-heeled as them, she could showcase the simple high-heeled boots, also made from calf leather, but sporting a round toe. The care card, branded dust bag and box are also included for a bargain £1,250.

The Bargain Bucket

Has anyone else noticed the carry-on at the reduced section in our supermarkets where shoppers can behave in the most bizarre fashion when confronted with bargain basement grub? In one well-known store, there were even reports of a tug of war between two eager bargain hunters – over a cut-price cucumber.

There are also ploys galore, so it seems, in order for peckish pests to get their mitts on the still-in-date cheap booty. One can strategically place one's child so other shoppers can't get to the low-price boiled beef and carrots, or just spread oneself around the vicinity trying to look bigger (like some bird species do) to ward off other hungry predators also out for a mosey. Then we have those types who pretend they are not interested in the rock-bottom swag because it's beneath them. They're perhaps the type who sneak bargain basement goodies into their basket when they think no one else is looking, to then duly hide the bright yellow reduced-price sticker under some expensive full-price dessert.

And what about those who pile all of the cut-price fodder into their trolley to the dismay and sometimes anger of the hovering pack? When poised at the reduced section, yours truly has been known to tut loudly when bearing witness to this underhand stroke. All's fair in war and scran, they could argue in retaliation.

Bargain Bucket-hungry shoppers should also be on their toes if their trolley is full to the wire with basement snips. If they were to inadvertently leave their low-price spoils while they rummage around for other steals, some mooching charlatan could pretend that they have mistaken their trolley for the reduced-price trolley and dip in. Now you wouldn't want that, would you? Especially if it results in a cat fight where one cannot now see the reduced section because of the clouded maelstrom of feline wisps.

It has also been documented that in one store, at approximately one hour before the cheap titbits go on sale, vulture-like scavengers circle the aisles ready to swoop. Then, as that clicking reduced-ticket machine-gun comes into view, salivating licking lips surge toward the treats.

Was that the noise of the gun dispensing those prized yellow tickets or was it a greedy hand being smacked because it's not quite reduction time? Then, just when one ravenous shopper thought they had bagged a giveaway jam roly-poly, an officious staff member's voice is heard above the melee.

"I've told you before – wait."

Yes, the Bargain Bucket squabbles might be all part of the fun for some hungry shoppers participating in the great supermarket scramble. In saying that, it's food for thought what would ensue if we were ever faced with a real-life food ration scenario.

On Being Human Prey

Having been lucky enough to go on safari at Kruger National Park in South Africa in 2012, my intellectual capacities expanded in line. The safaris were out of this world, where many things were learnt. The biggest lesson to be learnt however was the feeling of being pursued; my life could have been in jeopardy.

It was not a feeling to relish.

I had disagreed with quite a few Australians while resident at the lodge near to Kruger, including a newly married couple who were a little rough around the edges.

I have suffered from of mild case of novahollandiaphobia ever since.

A reasonable question was posed on one safari, in that because the wildlife industry is such a lucrative business, what would happen if a herd of animals, say, the wildebeest, migrated over the border from South Africa to Mozambique and remained. Would Mozambique then join the safari industry just to collect the revenue from tourists viewing the animals on their patch? It was a logical and interesting question, which was derided by the rather dim-witted Australian couple who, because they could not engage, made jokes about the animals getting passports and suchlike.

Even so, the smirks would be wiped from their scruffy faces soon after.

I enjoy asking far-reaching questions and the rangers (or tour guides) nearly always welcome the opportunity to divulge their knowledge. While viewing the lions, I got to thinking about the difference between sexes of all the animal kingdom (including human beings) and wondered why the female lion does most of the hunting with the male lion then commanding the kill. It was then that the male lion's roar was discussed. We concluded that the roar is an all-powerful signal to remind the rest of animal kind who is king of the jungle. In other words, the male lion has the valuable role of protecting the female from other beasts by possessing a deterrent that she does not possess herself. It was also debated why some animals are grass eaters (herbivores) and some meat eaters (carnivores) and how their teeth had evolved over millions of years to tally with available food sources. The changing landscape in relation to available food sustenance was also discussed, such as why a lion cannot survive without meat, but a large and powerful buffalo can. I determined that animals that eat both vegetation and meat (omnivores) have the best chance of surviving long-term.

Nonetheless, it was on the way home to the lodge, where ourselves and other tourists were staying, that the biggest and most important socio-educational quandary would present. All of a sudden, a red car with the windows blacked out began to follow us on the, by now, deserted road. Intermittently, ophidian menacing faces would lurk and loll out of the darkened glass apertures.

They were not playing a game of 'Peepo'.

Personally thinking, I just hoped that the female ranger who was driving carried a piece in her dash; I was perched in the front passenger seat, and the ignorant Australian couple were in the rear. I had heard the stories regarding tourists in South Africa getting shot dead for the price of a pair of trainers.

The car kept on trailing us and it was a surreal occurrence to know how it felt to be human prey. We then neared the site (lodge), at which the ranger quickly stated very seriously, what should we do: either carry on past the site, not letting the pursuers (or some would say hunters) know where we were staying, or turn in?

If you were faced with this dilemma, what would you do?

Of course I replied within a split second, animal instinct having taken over, this new-found cunning enabled me to state with conviction,

"Turn onto the site."

The reasons for this decision are as follows. If we had carried on, like prey in the jungle, we could have been isolated and/or backed into a corner which would have indeed lowered our chances of survival. On the other hand, if we turned on to our site, and as a result the trackers followed us in, just like the impala, there would be more victims for the assailants to choose from, some, I hate to add, perhaps weaker than us. There was safety in numbers. There could have been another armed ranger on duty at the lodge too, which would have also increased our survival chances.

The Australians sort of looked at me in a different way after that experience. The pursuers in the red car did not escalate their attack on that occasion and more than likely changed course to seek out easier kill.

Egg on the Face of First Buses

It's no fun travelling on First Bus in and around North Staffordshire. In between buses is the worst, as in when you alight from one and board another. It is at this point that you become very aware of the dangerous levels of pollution from vehicle emissions that First are greatly contributing to.

More worryingly, nobody seems to want to do anything about it. There are no long-term or even short-term strategies in place to offset this toxic situation by government or any other applicable authority.

I first raised the matter regarding the choking fumes from buses in general (especially those stationary and leaving their engines running) in the letters page of my local paper some ten years back and still nothing has changed. I think the letter was called *'Get your gas masks, it's First Buses'*. The correspondence seriously discussed the levels of pollution in the area and the detrimental health effects. I don't need a fancy technical measuring device or heed to weasel words from government appointed text-book boffins to gauge local contaminants, I taste them on a daily basis.

Furthermore, the 'new' routes adopted by First were the standing joke of the year. Now, when travelling on the 4A from Newcastle bus station to the town of Kidsgrove in the same borough (which takes forty-five minutes; yes it does not take that much longer to fly to Paris), the bus seems to go out of its way to make the journey longer. Instead of travelling straight to Knutton Lane roundabout en route to Sainsbury's, then on to Liverpool Road, for some strange unknown reason the bus turns along Merrial Street, then slowly meanders in the wrong direction down Church Street to turn back on itself up Lower Street and then on to Knutton Lane roundabout.

The bus never picks up any extra passengers by making this detour, either.

This is just one example of the absurd public transport routing system we have in place. There are lots more.

Another associated First irritant can be when passengers have waited a good while for a bus to arrive in the bus station only to be forced to linger another ten to fifteen minutes while the drivers change over.

The worst insult, however, is when the bus just becomes stationary at a stop; obviously because of timing. To sit there like muppets can be infuriating. Recently, during one journey on the number 25 from Newcastle to Hanley the bus actioned this manoeuvre of becoming static twice on the same trip. The second time it occurred (this time outside Stoke station) I enquired of the driver ever so matter-of-factly, "Are we going to sit here for another ten minutes like we have just done in Stoke town, mate?"

That quip got the bus moving. Believe me, I have had some run-ins over the years with the more ignorant of the bus drivers. On the contrary, in fairness to the company and to balance the argument, First can provide free onboard entertainment.

On one occasion, while travelling on the 4A through Chesterton, a loud thud was heard against the window.

"Jesus." I gasped, not knowing what it was.

Some kids had thrown an egg at the bus window and then run away.

One young girl from a group sitting at the back declared very maturely, "What was the point of that?"

Then a middle-aged female passenger got on her mobile phone.

"A told yer a don't like buzzees," she groaned down the handset.

"Theeve just thrown an egg at the winnder and run off."

At this point I was feeling a little sheepish in light of the young girl's comment. You see, as a kid in the early 1970s I used to throw eggs at buses in the Waterloo Road area of Hanley. We lobbed water-filled balloons at the buses too.

And what was the point of the egg throwing all those years ago?

Well, at the time I thought it was a laugh. I certainly wouldn't waste a good egg on First now, even though some would argue they would deserve it. Besides, they would only put their fares up again to pay for cleaning the window.

I tried to imagine the conversation amongst the driver and passengers on the old PMT bus after I had splattered an egg at the window all those years ago.

"Am telleen yer mother," would have been the shrill shriek from middle- to old-aged Elsie standing up to remonstrate at the bus window, as the vehicle shuddered to the stop.

I can almost see her sitting back down in her seat just as the bus started to move off again.

"Thee want a good hiding," I heard the bus driver chime, in a deep Potteries drawl.

"Ah blame the parents."

"It's that Keveen Rakkety from Trafalgar Street, he's notheen but trouble," Elsie chuntered to Flossie, an old lady sat next to her on the bus.

"Oooooh," replied Flossie.

Flossie acknowledged Elsie's statement with an Oooooh sound, beginning with an O for orange tone, a sort of Oooooh.

Flossie then adjusted her brown and orange flowery rustic-looking scarf, those old-fashioned ones that tie under the chin.

"A saw eem smokeen last week, he's a right little gangster up and down," Elsie added.

"Oooooh," said Flossie again.

Flossie emitted a louder and longer Oooooh every time Elsie reeled off, one by one, more of my misdemeanours. In fact, when Elsie had relayed the fact that I had smashed a window with a brick (in an old house by the way) then thrown a banger through it, Flossie's last Oooooh had reached a piercing crescendo.

"Ooooooooooooooooooooooooooooooooooh."

Yes, one has to have a fertile imagination while travelling with First Bus. The journeys take so long; a full novella can be scripted on the Newcastle-Hanley route.

The Spinning Jenny

Prime Minister Theresa May's 'speech' at the Conservative Party conference, Manchester, in October 2017, threw out some interesting self-punitive metaphors. To me, Calamity Jane's catastrophes were brought about because of raw poetic justice, no more, no less.

She did lieth and she did spin, didn't she? No wonder her voice deserted her in her hour of need.

Some of the more opinionated would emphatically declare that the letters falling off the set wall signified the falling apart of the Conservative Party; the meaning being that their political strap-line props are not as solid as they used to be. Regardless, according to the journalistic vanguards of the left, the *Guardian*: "It was, in fact, quite a good speech; an interesting one with some significant content. But that was lost amid the disruptions that overshadowed it."

I would refute this credence given to the Tories by our 'Leftist Literati'. Perhaps they also fancy themselves as comedians, on parallel lines with the joker who breached the stage. I find that generally, people who purposely try to raise laughs are not amusing in the grand comedic scheme of things. The funniest comedians are those who are not aware that they are entertaining; you can find many such comics in ordinary working-class life if anyone should care to look. Handing Theresa May her P45 was not comical at all, especially as it put straw-wigged Batty Boris in the spotlight once again.

Now he's enough to make a cat laugh; especially when filmed 'jogging' around the conference centre in short jodhpurs reminiscent of granny's blue floral curtains. He looked barmier than ever in his running attire, didn't he?

The most important symbolism attributed to the calamitous Ms May on the day in question, however, was losing her voice at significant intervals. Keeping in mind what was about to come out of her mouth, would we therefore conclude that the frog in her throat materialising at specific intervals during the oration was retributive justice of the vocalising kind?

With regard to her speech at conference, May stated that the NHS was world class and there would be an expansion of doctors and nurses where the Tories would always support high quality care. The cadence of her voice began to lose at this moment; I wonder why?

The prime minister's voice faltered yet again; this time when she was just about to declare that,

"We have created a record number of jobs." (She took a huge gulp of water after that verbal incongruity).

In reality, the majority of the new jobs created are unskilled and low paid, verging on slave labour, where zero-hour contracts are commonplace and the majority of working people struggle to survive.

May then added that,

"We would not hesitate to act if businesses aren't operating as they should."

This mis-statement saw the prime minister's voice trail into a servile whimper. Perhaps it was because she knew and we knew it was one of the biggest boggers of all. Big business has just about got away with every worker atrocity in the book. Under guidance stemming from Tory ideology, we have seen companies streamlining, price hiking, over profiteering and shifting the onus on the customer to fulfil corporate obligations as outlined in another article. Then we have the shoddy, unprofessional manner some businesses operate when dealing with the public; such as cutting quality to maximise profit.

In between splutters, the prime minister also fancied herself as a bit of a comedienne. After the delaying tactic of receiving a cough sweet from Chancellor Philip Hammond, she cracked the unfunniest jokes of the year. One ditty being: "Ladies and gentlemen, look at the Chancellor giving something away for free." The ripostes were hardly Oscar Wilde territory, were they? Even so, we saw plenty of false smiles and guffaws (teeth and all) emanating from the contrived audience of Conservative Party colleagues who were sensing a PR disaster of gargantuan proportions.

Mealy-mouthed May's voice also faltered when she began to expand on Manchester's great industrial past (the Industrial Revolution of the late

1700s mid-1800s) as if the period was something to be proud about. She proclaimed that:

"Cities like Manchester were the pioneers that fired the Industrial Revolution, helping to make Britain the workshop of the world."

In reality, during this period, it was children in the cotton mills of Lancashire living a purgatorial existence that helped make Britain the sweatshop, not workshop, of the world. Children were favoured by unscrupulous factory owners because they worked for less pay and had smaller, more nimble fingers for 'piecing' which consisted of tying loose cotton under heavy machinery. Children were also useful commodities because they could crawl more easily under the heavy and dangerous equipment, where the child's loose clothing and hair could be entangled, resulting in serious injury like losing a limb. Children of that era would start a twelve-hour day in the mills as young as four. If they did not suffer mill-related diseases or cancers, these children could in fact be killed on the factory floor, sometimes through scavenging (cleaning out machinery while it was still running) or falling asleep over the cotton-making apparatus due to severe exhaustion because of overwork.

Addiction and
the Artist's Impression

Post-Impressionist Vincent van Gogh (1853–1890) used the colour yellow in many of his paintings. Yet, this was not necessarily down to his love of the colour, or even a response to a psychedelic experience from ingesting mind-altering substances. It was more than likely because of his jaundice and yellow vision brought on by absinthe abuse. What can also be discussed is the idea that *The Potato Eaters* (1885) mirrors Van Gogh's own shadowy gloom, pertaining directly to his mental state at the time.

The question that is being posed in the addiction school of thought today is whether substances can open the creative mind, in that those who are predisposed to original creation can produce inconceivable works of art under the influence of a substance.

Let's first of all look at some of the artistic greats. It is believed that Lewis Carroll liked the 'Wonderland' effects of magic mushrooms, the Beatles used marijuana and LSD, and Edgar Allan Poe's dark, disturbed and depressed mind fed on opium and alcohol.

Some artistic types have also described the 'eureka moment' of coming up with that mind-blowing storyline, a novel brushstroke perspective, or even a cutting-edge song title after being affected by drugs.

But was it really attributed to the substances they had consumed, or could it be that the mood is so exaggerated by substances to such an extent that this eureka moment, when taken apart in the cold light of day, is pretty intangible and unassuming?

Likewise, if one did come up with an extremely novel idea under the influence, who could say that they would not have come up with the same idea when completely sober? As in when sober of thought, the artist's new ideas could be so mundane, matter of fact and conventional in the everyday mindset of the artist, that those ideas do not warrant any profound pronunciation.

Great minds apart, the practicalities for those in addiction can see mental health problems arising and progressing simultaneously with that of the habit. This can be exemplified by Vincent van Gogh. Let's face it; to cut off your own ear is not a sign of mental stability. When van Gogh entered the asylum in 1889, his paintings thereafter took on a definitive and distinct 'mad twinge' about them. How strange.

There is another argument that drugs can tear down the barriers of convention and allow one to delve into different surreal dimensions. This is perhaps true, but it would be delusional to think that these dimensions necessarily equate to great artistic expression.

Then there is the notion that great art can be produced while psychotic or schizophrenic (which artistic addicts will no doubt be suffering from after prolonged use of a substance). This might be the case because there is a fine line between genius and madness. Nevertheless, it is too great a risk to push the mind into unknown territory for the sake of one's art. It is possible that after one such artistic excursion into the abyss, one might not quite return to complete their 'masterpiece'.

To polish up one's art and consistently reproduce over long periods, then to painstakingly correct and redraft to get your finished product ready for distribution is laborious. What's more, to have the confidence to sell that work of art in the marketplace is a task that cannot be achieved while under the influence.

The Battle for Britain

There has always been an interest in corresponding one's birth month with that of a famous person. But what about going one further and corresponding one's birth town with the appropriate notable figure too?

Well, I was lucky enough to have arrived on this earth in the town of Kidsgrove in the month of May, which corresponds with that of our very own Reginald Mitchell. Born on Congleton Road, Butt Lane, Kidsgrove, in the borough of Newcastle-under-Lyme and educated at Hanley High, Reginald Mitchell (1895–1937) is perhaps North Staffordshire's most famous son.

Although the first prototype Spitfire, serial K5054, flew for the first time on the 5th March 1936 at Eastleigh in Hampshire, sadly Reginald Mitchell did not live long enough to witness his famous aircraft take the central role in the Battle of Britain (began July 10th 1940 and lasted three and a half months). He died in 1937 aged just forty-two.

Did you know that the Potteries Museum and Art Gallery in Hanley displays the Spitfire (years ago the same aircraft used to be exhibited in a glass case opposite the museum)?

In fact our aeronautical engineer and his accomplishments are the main focal point exhibits that even surpass the Staffordshire Hoard on the interest scale. Notwithstanding, with the 75th anniversary of the definitive World War 2 Battle of Britain just passed, can some thought-provoking modern-day comparisons be drawn? As in, could we speculate that there are comparable ideological battles currently going on in the Labour Party similar to those battles between Britain and Germany during the war?

Perhaps those who yearn for a fairer political, social and cultural structure to displace the tired and overworked current order are analogous to that of Great Britain and those who aspire to the existing 'greed is good' mantra (the Conservative Party and their Tory Lite allies in the Labour Party) are comparable to Germany.

In reference to Germany's allies; UKIP could be cast as totalitarian Japan (although in fairness, it was UKIP who harvested the Brexit vote) and the 'go along with the anything for power', Lib Dems pitched as Italy to keep with the WW2 idea.

The Battle of Britain analogy would also have to refer to the Rules of Engagement, especially with regard to Germany (or the Conservative and Labour-Tory-Lites). During the race for the Labour leadership in 2015, their tactics were anything but honourable.

We saw the double bluff nonsense in that many Tories had joined the Labour Party just to vote for Corbyn (or a like principled figure) to peddle the fiction that if he got elected, the Labour Party would never be voted into government again.

Talk about psychological warfare. The real truth of the matter is that the Conservative and the Labour-Tory-Lites do not want the system to change in any way, shape, or form at any cost. This is because that same established order capitalises handsomely from the current selfish unequal status quo. Subsequently, their real fear is that an ordinary people-led movement will gradually gain credence and supersede the Conservatives as the main political force in Britain. Then we have that other reprehensible fallacy that to initiate a new direction for the Labour Party would result in a disastrous loss as seen in the 1983 general election.

Many would argue that it is impossible to draw this distinction, being that the 1983 election was held over thirty years ago in a completely different macroclimate than that of today.

Yes, one can safely argue that the Spitfire Exhibition at our brilliant Potteries Museum and Art Gallery has significance in the grand political scheme of things.

Those who wish for radical change advocate greater investment in the environment, health, education, transport, business and, of course, cultural institutions like museums and libraries which will require consistent financial outlay to maintain.

Today's modern man (us) will be known to posterity in thousands of years hence as an ancient civilisation. Perhaps in this futuristic society, visitors to establishments like the Potteries Museum will hold their hands over their mouths in shock on witnessing the 2015 Foodbank Exhibition depicting what a working family would have to survive on for a whole week.

Returning to the Battle of Britain analogy, in 2015, Britain, (or the new movement) won the Labour Party trajectory battle. But can they win the next General Election War?

The Blurring of the Lines

There are those abroad who mock the weather in Britain as if we are partly responsible for the natural climatic patterns. In saying that, the British weather can be an interesting spectacle when our skies produce contrasting variegated blushes of greys, blues and blacks instead of the sheet of sky blue every hour of every day. We can also experience fluid and shifting spasms of rain, wind (that can sometimes cut into the face) sun and even snow, all in the space of a short interval. It's true to say that the Lake District in Cumbria always conforms to our predictable weather arrangement orthodoxy.

Weather shifting; if one should Google 'How old is Lake Windermere' one would discover a few differing results. In other words, we don't know. I would hazard a guess at a few million (years old that is). Some say the 10.5-mile lake was formed 13,000 years ago in the advent of the last major ice age occurring in England.

It was decided to visit the Lake District in November when the multitudes of tourists had abated, although it must also be said that during this time, the local bus service abates too. Trains, buses, the odd taxi and good old-fashioned foot slogging (walking) will enable you to cover some ground. Kendal (Cumbria) is also a practical and accessible gateway to the southern Lake District region.

While in this locality, the Beatrix Potter Museum in Bowness-on-Windermere is well worth a visit, even if, like me, you tend to be a little cynical regarding the middle-class-Milly animal character names such as, Flopsy, Mopsy and Cotton Tail (which tend to sound a little silly and outdated by today's standards). Whatever the animal names; animation tales are always great fun. Plus, only by visiting the museum can the more scathing amongst us learn how Helen Beatrix Potter became such a successful story writer. The fact that her grandfather owned the largest printing press in England at the time had nothing to do with it, of course.

Beatrix aside, my final day in the Lake District would provide some unusual entertainment considering that I had decided to embark on a boat excursion around Lake Windermere. While chatting with the receptionist at the hotel in Kendal and asking about the illustrious body of water, I seriously enquired if there were any speedboats at the lakeside to trip out on. The receptionist then sort of smirked when disclosing the fact that there were speed restrictions in place on the lake.

It was still dark and lightly drizzling on that particular morning when I boarded the bus to Windermere. Speedboat indeed. Perhaps the receptionist thought I fancied myself as a bit of a James Bond type, starring in *The Man on the Icy Lake*. She probably envisaged me determined to spin around the lakes in a series of jump cuts (an abrupt transition from one scene to another) at 100 miles per hour, to the astonishment and amusement of locals and tourists alike.

How boring, I dwelt. What was wrong with a quick and rapid whizz around the waterway?

"This is my country too; why can't I have a say in what we can and cannot do?"

Forget the English sonnet; what was being analysed at this moment in time was how we are being controlled. Did some jumped-up councillor 'on Committeh' (the committee) introduce the speed-limit ruling to demonstrate their little bit of authority? It was on this notion that I went into James Bond mode and pondered if a 007 storyline had ever included the famous secret agent flashing his concessionary bus pass as he boarded the bus to Bowness (Scaramanga would never have kopped on to that one it was quickly identified).

It would be a beguiling, mesmerising environmental Bond feature, filmed partly in the Lake District with its millions-of-years-old lakes as an appropriate set. James would be saving the world from an environmental disaster to the detriment of our very own double agent Constants Moneypacker, but the modern 'packing it in' auteurs know best, you know.

Back to reality on the portside of Windermere, the first two cruises were cancelled because of the imposing fog. I waited petulantly.

A kind of slow steamer was then boarded which would steer me around the former glaciers. One port of recall was Ambleside. The picture was reminiscent of what the great English portrait artists would have frescoed; the odd and the opaquely demure, with that suggestion of the enigmatic smear.

As I perused the lake, the horizon and the murky sky became blurred, making the vista not quite right. In that there was no defining line to determine the sky and the waterline. It had all merged into one.

The fog thickened.

The M.O. of the Mosquito

After reading the story of the lady who was hospitalised after a mosquito bite, it moved me to tell a true story of my own regarding these horrific insects. More deadly than any venomous snake or rabid tiger, to have a battle with the mosquito is one you are never likely to forget. This resourceful creature kills some 500,000 people every year, with another 200 million people incapacitated because of being bitten. The mosquito also threatens half of the world's population and causes billions of pounds in lost productivity. Other mosquito-related diseases include dengue fever, yellow fever, and encephalitis. Last but not least, their saliva contains anaesthetic properties, so you don't feel the little b*****ds drawing your blood…

The nightmare for me started with a steamy hot night in Crete where muggins here had unwittingly thrown all the windows open to invite them in for their liquid dinner (they must have thought mosquito Christmas had come early). I had never been bitten before. The very next morning I found that I had red lumps all over my face including my nose, ears and shoulders; the bites quickly turned yellow and I sought advice.

After rubbing cream into my wounds, I began to decode how to gain the upper hand against the midges and reckoned that they had better get up early to catch me out again (not realising that dawn was their most active time of day).

I bought lotions and potions and even one of those smoky whirlygigs could be seen emanating fumes from my room 200 yards away. I love nature I calculated, but it was now a personal battle and it was me or them and I knew that I was facing a determined enemy.

One was spotted on the wall briefly, or in my mosquito-induced delirium was it a black spot before my very eyes? I let rip with a tea towel and yes, it was my blood spattered over the wall.

I had scored a direct hit.

Think strategically, I rationalised, like a general at war against formidable opposition. All the windows were then methodically sealed as the room was given a good gassing in anticipation of the next night approaching… would they launch another attack I deciphered, checking under the sheets in case one of the bleeders had plans for me to sleep with the enemy.

The moral to this story is; give the varmints an inch of your flesh and they will take not a mile but bite you to death and show no mercy when doing so. Mosquitoes can display a dogged determination unparalleled in the animal kingdom as they lure you into traps and false senses of security you never believed possible. You can actually think you have beaten them only to be reminded with a buzz in your ear the very next night that they are no pushover. Those who become complacent because they don't usually get bitten think again – as we speak a new mutant of mosquito is probably in metamorphosis.

I learnt to respect the mosquito the hard way.

Trick Photography in Lunarote

There are some compensations for getting older. Instead of rotting in bed sleeping off the booze you can instead bear witness to the delights of dawn over the coast of North Africa (Lanzarote in this case) from the hotel veranda.

Next stop Western Sahara.

Talking of which, the hot Saharan squalls that sweep over to Lanzarote from the desert can literally whisk you off your feet in exhaustion, from where only copious amounts of water drinking will bring you round.

I like Lanzarote; sun all year round and the extremely curious volcanic environment where the lava landscape, torn and etched out through years of pounding from the sea, delights spectacularly.

If you like snorkelling don't forget to take some bread with you. Those cheeky striped fish will follow you all day for a morsel, but don't go too far out, although the stripy fish aren't piranha-esque. I would reckon a shoal of them would chance their arm if you went out too far and there was no bread for them to swipe. As in they may start nibbling at you instead.

Timanfaya National Park or Fire Mountain is a must to see. There are still active volcanoes in the park where one can cook chickens from the volcanic heat to eat in the restaurant.

This volcanic, lunar-like landscape allows one to feel that you are, in fact, in outer space.

Come on, jokes aside, those Yanks no more landed on the moon in 1969 than the man in the moon. I don't do conspiracy theories myself, but those astronauts had to be Hollywood stuntmen bouncing up and down in space suits in the darkly-lit lunar landscape of Lanzarote. For me this logical theory was reinforced when I caught sight of a NASA bunker at Timanfaya the first time I had visited. The Americans are expert at trick photography, especially when engaging in psychological warfare with the USSR/Russia. When I took a photograph of one area which was most lunar-like, the flash caught on the bus window and made it appear as though the light could have been an unexplained UFO in the distance.

I learnt all about perspectives at university.

The Green Lagoon area in Lanzarote is also well worth a visit, how strange a landscape is that, you might ask?

Surely it's not going to be referred to in the future as Mars or Jupiter, we ain't that daft across the pond you know.

Karma – I'll have you off; you have me off

Karma is a phenomenon found in Indian religions (Hinduism and Buddhism, for example) which in Sanskrit translates to the fact that the action or deed causes the cycle of cause and effect.

In other words, what goes around comes around (and vice versa).

Warped or negative karma is the thinking/action that if you should lose something and nobody hands it in, it would be justifiable that you should then keep and not hand in anything you should find.

Some are cynical regarding karma, as in they argue that many tread on another for their own personal or monetary gain and nothing untoward seems to happen to them.

This may be the case.

To bring karma into the modern-day perspective I lost/left my treasured and relatively expensive personal CD player on the bus and nobody handed it in.

A few weeks later, on another bus, I found an expensive mobile telephone and immediately handed it to the, by now, frantic teenager searching around for it.

If I was that way inclined, I could have easily slipped it in my pocket.

The teenager thanked me profusely, exclaiming that "My mum would have killed me". It has to be the right thing to do; to hand back another's property, that is.

But what is the conservative estimate in our modern-day culture regarding who would hand in a lost item and who would not – fifty/fifty, maybe?

Older people are more likely (one supposes) to hand in a lost/found item.

Then why, do you imagine, some people keep property that does not belong to them, and what does stealing by finding say about the society that we live in?

What is known, is that if you do a good turn for another, a good turn has more chance of coming back to you in return.

Well, let's look at the law of karma in the aforementioned case. Having lost the personal CD player it could have been reasoned by some that the found mobile telephone was compensation for the lost/stolen CD player; as it evened the scores (I should have kept the device).

No thank you, I don't want to live in a society governed by the 'I'll have you off; you have me off' warped and negative sense of karma.

Perhaps I broke a destructive cycle.

Pre-Ramble

In 2015 I visited Portcullis House in Westminster to attend a seminar on homelessness. Opened in 2001, the facility was initiated to house MPs and their staff to supplement the limited space in the nearby Palace of Westminster. The rooms inside this Westminster add-on include, amongst many others, the Thatcher Room, the Wilson Room and the Attlee Room. Still, austerity does not seem to apply here. More than £500,000 of taxpayers' money was to be spent sprucing up Portcullis House, with £144,000 earmarked for wood lacquering and another £180,000 for fixtures and fittings. This work includes decorating as well as specialist wallpapers, not forgetting, of course, that another £40,000 is needed to tend to twelve fig trees flowering there.

When visiting London in the past, I would always end up at Westminster for some strange reason, remembering that there are only so many times one can marvel at the statue of Boudica and her chariot.

This time around, I assumed the persona of the 'know-where-they-are-going' type which is a personality foible in the human condition that can be irritating, to say the least. Marching hitherto, similarly instructing colleagues to "follow me" even though they had hinted we were going in the wrong direction, I took us to the entrance of the Houses of Parliament instead.

Not really wanting to admit I had got it wrong I mitigated instead that my co-worker/s should have spoken up louder if they had known the directions.

Lesson learnt for me. Enough of the preamble, let's get to the crux of the piece. Not ones for learning lessons, sitting MPs who participate in forums, events, meetings and discussions still seem to believe that this platform is a cue for them to ramble on for some thirty minutes or more. Usually uttering empty rhetoric of what is happening with regard to the homeless in this example.

Yes, it was painful having to sit through it.

When we eventually came to questions at the end of the event, and not one for beating about the bush, I asked the political 'panel' in so many words: in light of the devastating effects austerity measures are having on the marginalised (with services closing down) and taking into consideration the fact the right honourable gentlemen wanted to help the homeless, would they be voting against austerity then?

Indubitably, it was a catch-22 question and of course they would be voting for austerity not against it, but at least the whole 'help the homeless' nonsense was put into context. One or two of the panel looked visibly ruffled when I stated, "That's a different argument" in response to one Tory MP intent on putting us through more meaningless and elongated diatribes regarding the plight of Greece and their subsequent austerity measures.

Yours truly was then ever so politely told off by the chair, whereby it was deduced that we could not respond to any statements made by the panel; but should allow those political representatives to drone on some more.

In other words, we could not participate in a democratic debate with fair exchanges. We had to be subjected to the *experts'* take on the subject and be thankful for it.

Yes, I am getting quite good at posing searching questions to the spin artists of this world, having now practiced my technique in a difficult arena (licking my lips as I write, wondering how my transparent queries can embarrass more of them).

These people need to be challenged.

The Truman Show

In introduction to this piece, I would like to bring the reader's attention to the desperate state our local institutions are in today. Firstly, with the sometimes incompetent/negligent/dangerous local councils, and secondly, with the appalling and bizarre methods employed by local police, just so the public can report crime. However, in making the police statement above, it has to be considered that nationally, police forces are facing unprecedented cuts to their budgets.

In August 2017, I got in a taxi from the rank outside the railway station. It was a bigger taxi than the others, but not like the big black taxis. I paid the fare of £6 outside my home and secured a receipt. Still, being exhausted, I went straight to bed and the next day, I realised my wallet had gone. After searching my flat just in case, I then went to the rank outside the station and asked around. I was told that the receipt was worthless and the driver could not be contacted via that same receipt. In my missing wallet were several forms of identity and bankcards, plus my business card with my contact telephone number. There was also £180–£200 in cash because I was about to pay the decorator.

This means that if there is a serious incident regarding a taxi, the taxi driver cannot be traced, which does not bode well in today's climate. The taxi rank is registered at the council by the licensing department which brings one to wonder why the council are allowing worthless receipts to be handed out unchecked. In fact, I am flabbergasted by this incompetence. Going through other receipts from the same rank, five more, over a three-month period, were also discovered to have meaningless squiggles which were supposed to be the names of the drivers who had taken fares.

I then decided to report the matter to the police, who are now stationed in the town hall, but I was told there were no police in attendance all week and would have to either telephone the 101 number, or use the grey intercom for contacting the police which was located outside in the street. Opting for the intercom, being wary that there could be a charge for the call, an irritated loud voice on the other end of loudspeaker, for the whole town to hear, bellowed out, "What crime are you reporting?" They then asked for my name and address which was also bawled out in loud decibels for all and sundry to hear. I was shocked and belittled; in fact this system of contact would deter people from reporting crime. It was then quickly decided to abort the 'intercom', opting for the 101 number instead.

A police constable then arrived who said one could report crimes at the civic centre. Having then made enquiries, you have to make an appointment to report a crime at the civic centre. In retrospect, the person who had eventually taken my call (101) said that the intercom system magnifies the voice, so it appears as though the call centre operatives are shouting. In addition, the staff at the town hall were in agreement that the intercom system is ridiculous.

I felt like I was taking part in some warped English variation of *The Truman Show*; especially when our local football club (I had season cards in the wallet), not the police, notified me two weeks later that my wallet had been found; even though the wallet had been handed into the police station.

European Regiment Para-mount

To put it bluntly, the current policy of free movement around Europe has been a catastrophic failure and has added to the current refugee crisis. This is the main reason Saint Angela of Germany took in so many migrants – to save face. That policy, however, will no doubt backfire.

As such, the call for a European Regiment is of paramount importance; our continent needs coordinated, sophisticated patrol from all European nations. Bearing in mind that frontiers with Asia and North Africa have been exposed as passive and penetrable as seen with the migrant mass exodus. Although a European army has been propagated as being unpopular here in Britain, some kind of special forces European military unit has to be commissioned sooner rather than later for strategic and security purposes. Britain or any other European country does not need to be inside the haemorrhaging EU to be part of this European defence system.

The facts of the matter are this. The migrant pandemonium as seen in Greece, Italy and Hungary is partly a result of interference by Europe and the US in Libya, Afghanistan, Iraq and Syria. To describe the West as destabilising the region is perhaps putting it mildly.

The US and Britain have also manipulated the ISIS/ISIL/IS (or whatever) presence as part of a general plan to dictate policy in the Middle East and we are now paying the price.

In 2017, the allied proposal was to repeatedly bomb IS out of Syria, so making it safe again. Have you ever heard anything so preposterous? What we really need is a statesman (or woman) with enough backbone to call all of the Middle Eastern/North African factions around the table with immediate effect. All wars come to an end; why not this one sooner rather than later?

I am sure the politically intelligent would agree that it's only by diplomacy that instability and warring can be resolved so we can enter into an era of world peace; military action has to be a last resort. We need open and direct lines of communication with Russia (what have they ever done to us; they were our allies during World War 2), China, Argentina and even North Korea, all of whom will negotiate. The process has already been initiated with the recent thawing of relations with Iran which the Conservatives and US President Obama can take some credit for.

Talking of Obama and now Trump, the British Isles need to build equal relationships with all the nations of the world. We don't want our country to cocoon itself inside a warped, one-sided, secretive and imperialistic bubble alongside the elites of Europe, the US, Saudi Arabia and Israel. But then again, as of July 2018, that special relationship Britain has had over the years with the US appears well and truly spent (especially with regard to the new US trade tariffs). Three cheers for this unexpected development.

For Europe to resume or initiate trade with many of the 'forgotten nations' of the world will boost business and our market economy to an unprecedented level. For those same nation-states (and the rest of the world) to bear witness to the fact that we are a peaceful, democratic, but security conscious continent, possessing a dynamic European army protecting our frontiers, can only propel proficient economic activity internationally for the benefit of all Europeans.

Squirrel Esquire and the Human Nuts

Once upon a time there existed a paradise called Squirreldom. It was perfection in every way where animal life marvelled at the natural balance. Basking in the utopian equilibrium lived many a squirrel, hopping gracefully, burying a nut or two. Long, long ago and longer ago than that, the squirrels lived on the land where Blacky the Blackbird and Maggie the Magpie venerated the nut antics from close distance. Squire Squirrel was one such graceful squirrel. He was a good and fair Sheriff of Squirreldom. The feathers in his brow had been deserved on many a brave and courageous occasion. He was fearless in every way. Yes, he possessed the largest nut cache, but he unselfishly shared all the nuts between the rest of the squirrel kingdom. He merited those Squirrelly feathers in that dapper, squirrelly cap.

He didn't 'even hog the biggest nuts for himself.

It had been a huge harvest day the last ideals of March and nuts had been in abundance. There had been glad tidings with a binding Squirrel ceremony by the Old Church Door. The meadow hummed.

"Smile," squawked Page Squirrel as he squatted to take photographic aim.

Nuts a-showered the eventing couple.

As the nuts rained down on the olde cobbled gravestones, audible tinkling sounds echoed in the little furry ears of the Squirrels on this beautiful squirrelly day. Drenched in happy sunlight, the heated climatic green bed of grass swayed to the balanced contentment.

Mrs Squirrelly said the very word with more of a "Hhm" as she made her entrance.

She even adorned the precious emerald clover neck chain that the Squire had devised her earlier at the engagement. They epitomised bliss. And so it would be for some years to pass in Happy Squirreldom.

UNTIL THE HUNTERS CAME.

Flash back: happy church door, turns into red and black at night.

Grim Grime nailing Page Squirrelly to the church door.

There would be a price paid for the spilt blood.

"Here's your ration," squeaked Squire Squirrel to Mrs Squirrelly.

"And an extra few for the new arrival," he chirped and chattered, with a nod and a wink in reference to Mrs Squirrelly's distended squirrelly bump affronting her soft squirrelly pelt.

Mrs Squirrelly appeared laden down with her nest of young squirrels in tow, tugging at her squirrelly squeaky clean apron strings. She did not know how she would make the nuts last the bleak and cold winter months. She twitched longingly towards the little squirrelly picture of her Squeaky first born. The kitten had been taken, she recalled, in the most brutal fashion. Mrs Squirrelly's little squirrelly voice almost broke.

"Many thanks, Squire Squirrel," squeaked Mrs Squirrelly in a faltering but composed voice. "They will come in handy for the trip to Nutsford."

She momentarily smiled and forgot the drudge of bringing up her little brood of squirrels alone. It had been difficult since the human hunters had murdered her devoted husband, the squadron leader of Squire Squirreldom.

She was now the main nut provider. The last squire of the pasture had been miserly. Half the squirrel neighbourhood delighted when he fled the countryside with the vicar's daughter. Married man, and all, she tutted, very squirrel-like, to herself.

It had been talk of the trees for weeks.

You could not say that the bonehead brothers Grime were animals. It would be an insult to the other species. They were more akin to fiends. The most hardy would be repulsed at their demeanours.

"Are we going hunting tonight?" belched Grim Grime, the older and grimier of the two brothers.

"Yeah, if you like," retorted the younger brother, Gruesum, the nastiest brute of the clan.

"Fancy squirrel meat for tea?" he added, belching and flatulating simultaneously. The two Grime brothers laughed very coarsely out loud. They were definitely the most brutish, gruesome creatures you ever did see.

Squire Squirrel nested down in his little oak tree. He had done his squirreling duties for the day and so nervously but deservedly, nibbled at a large-looking nut that he had kept for his supper. He knew in his little squirrel heart that the hunters were due.

"Why couldn't they just leave us alone to do our squirreling?" he squirreled out loud. With this squirrely sentiment Squire Squirrel curled up his little squirreled bushy tail and began drifting off into squirrelly slumber.

Bang

Mrs Squirrelly squealed very squirrel-like and woke up the whole neighbourhood doing so. Pandemonium ensued. Squire Squirrel squirmed with dread. He had heard that caterwaul before. A few squirrels were massacred and mutilated, that fateful night in question, he remembered last.

The mess was crimsoned grey.

There would be distasteful retribution for the squirrels in a future occurrence.

But new laws would be passed in the land making squirrel hunting a serious offence.

The bullyboy Grime brothers would rue the day they ever set foot in Squirreldom. A celebration melody emanated from the household thereafter the slaughter. The unwanted residents were about to celebrate not with nuance, but with the graver charge of aggravated nuisance. Squirrel Pie was on Ma Grime's menu. Tea-stained home-sweet-home pictures decorated the wall and noxious smoke riddled the air.

Gruesum was not about to be in celebration mood, though. He would face head-on in horror his impending dearth.

And would sensate every sequence.

Party night it was called at the Grimes Grimiest of Grottos. An intense urinary odour suffocated the senses and drenched every demise. One of the brothers' base chums, named Grotty, made coarse chewing sounds amid wiping her snout repulsively in between takes. Debauched drunken revelry of the lowest kind was about to erupt.

Gruesum waddled his hips jack-assily; in some sort of absurd mating ritual. All in a ridiculous pitiful attempt to attract Grotto's young sister Grossie, the gross lump of fat lard sat yonder.

It was at that time that Grossie had plummeted her grubby fingers into the bowl of peanuts doled out by Gruesum's very Gruelly-looking obese mother, Gruella Grime, who, at this time, was gratuitously gruelling her unclean face with nourishment. Her ugly boat-race almost blushed salmon pink, reflected in the silver salted nut bowl in between her black fingernailed claws as she excavated nuts. She wiggled her unkempt long mop of dirty slimed hair. One strand had strayed in the dank air to land in Grim's tankard of rough cider. He picked it out and sucked on it.

It would be the hairs on Gruesum's back that were about to stand on end in terror during this equation.

In his sheer gluttony, Gruesum unearthed the biggest handful of nuts ever scooped. He pathetically and simultaneously glared drunkenly in stupid base hope at some insignificant digits.

"D'ya know what I'm going to do when I win the lottery?" he garbled in drunken-based overtones. His ludicrous party piece had plummeted to depths unmentionable.

Gruesum's talk spittle was thrown over quite a distance where it nestled on some once white, but now dirty black, pinafore dress; whence the bearer, would not even bat an oblivious eyelid.

He was the most boorish of all specimens known to mankind, alive or otherwise, was Gruesum.

It was somewhere around this stage that Gruesum facilitated that the face of the devil was perilously close. Horrific darkness clasped a black macabre which enveloped Gruesum Grime with force. His psyche popped out of the brainicular in a choking movement that one could only call sheer abyss. Physicalities then stated he shone a deathly white blewy hue as he rasped his last breath. Gruesum begged not to perish but his pleas were in vain. Then a sort of deranged and lunatic shriek emanated the Grime residence.

Ma Grime flung her flea-ridden dirty heavy body over her dead and debilitated son.

And the silly large oaf triggered 'shotgun' loaded by the grimmer Grim Grime at a previous bash. The wounds from the projectile abounded the coarse laggard's face. The earth shuddered as her colossal frame hit the deck. Thunder and frightening ensued.

In the most repugnant of shocks, the evil Gruesum Grime would depart his stinking earth.

And worse still, Grim Grime, the younger brother, would never get over it.

Nails tore right through his hands as he slumped down the olde church door in one pathetic heap. Grim had been playing for very high stakes and had miscarried miserably.

The last time seen he could be heard rambling incoherently, alone and wasted. Grim spent the remainder of his degenerate days as a vagrant, permanently fused with every narcotic imaginable, disturbed by intrusions of psychotic nuts.

"Please can you help me, sir?" whined Grim Grime in pleading syllables.

He had ended up where he was born and belonged, in the gutter.

Purple and black track marks were visible through veined spindled fissures – green and yellow mucous dribbled inconsistently. Yes, Grim Grime had got it bad. His pitiful life, that is.

A startled passer-by hurried their pace as the wretched sky opened up. The rain pelted relentlessly and the north wind icy blue.

What went around came around for the brothers Grime.

The Immigration Debate

Although immigration is a topical and serious issue in politics today, one cannot help but despair at how the mainstream parties play cheap party politics around the status of the immigrant.

My personal views on immigration have always been very clear. The doors to our country need to be closed with immediate effect and resources used to investigate fully those who are domiciled here illegally.

In addition, it can be argued that in some communities the different ethnic mix has proved fractious in as much as it has been suggested that some immigrants in our country set themselves apart by language and cultural practices. In other words, they don't integrate.

In saying this, Newcastle-under-Lyme does not have a serious immigration problem and if we had, as a civilised people, we do not want to orchestrate a witch hunt against others of a different nationality/culture. Many of us hold the virtues of kindness, fairness, diversity and civility in our own national traits, insomuch as we do not want immigrants to feel demonised or victimised because of ethnic or cultural differences. It also goes without saying that if more immigrants were to enter the country, such would be the civil unrest it would destabilise and compromise the migrants already settled.

It can be safely said that the blame for the influx of the immigrant lies with ruthless big business owners (backed by government) who strive for cheap labour at the expense of our own indigenous workforce, whose pay and conditions are driven down as a result. This is characterised by employment agencies touting for cheap labour overseas where they infiltrate foreign job markets to lure desperately poor people to relocate to our shores.

One does suppose though that we would do exactly the same if we found ourselves in that desperate position and, historically speaking, we have done (emigration to North America and Australia, for example).

We should also remember, of course, that originally the Anglo-Saxons were invading immigrants from Central and Eastern Europe.

Inquiry into Enquiries

After meticulously crafting my mother's death notice for a local newspaper on Friday the 6th of January 2017 (without any mistakes) I emailed it to the funeral directors, who then emailed it to the paper. I later noticed an error in the proof of the notice which said 'inquiries' should be made to the funeral director, instead of 'enquiries' should be made to the funeral director. After researching the words, in Britain the word inquiry is used if there is to be an investigation of sorts. In the USA, the word inquiry is used for both an investigation and in asking for something. It should be emphasised that we are in Britain not the US, so technically speaking this is an error. Use of the word inquiries instead of enquiries suggest that British institutions are allowing our language to slowly erode in favour of US-style colloquialisms.

I rang the paper overseer several times, but they were closed and did not leave any contact number for bereaved and distressed relatives should incidents like this occur over the weekend. On the Saturday morning I emailed them and requested the death notice not be published in the 'inquiries' for 'enquiries' format.

On the Monday morning (9th January 2017) I looked on the newspaper's website obituary notices and saw that the spelling had not been changed – the notice read inquiries instead of enquiries. I then wrote to them and stated to the effect that the misspelling suggested the staff were not exercising due care and diligence at such a sensitive time for grieving relatives. I also went on to say that the family were very angry at this because the word enquiries was spelled perfectly when the death notice was sent via email, which suggests that someone had meddled unnecessarily with it. I reiterated the point that this was about basic grammar, which all professional companies should have a handle on, and also relayed that nonsensical or incorrect grammar as seen in a death notice is poor presentation, which conveys a tacky message at such a delicate time. I felt that my mother's passing had been rubbished. I also made the point that there was no emergency contact number over the weekend.

Approximately two hours later 'inquiries' had been changed to 'enquiries' in my mother's death notice on the website.

The funeral director then telephoned me and told me that the newspaper had telephoned him and apologised and agreed to refund the £100 fee for the death notice as compensation. I later received an email from the publication who admitted that it was indeed a spelling mistake; they wrote:

Good morning Mr Raftery,

Thank you for your e-mails regarding the error in the notice for your late mother. I would firstly like to take this opportunity to apologise for the error made in the notice.

I have now been able to investigate the issue and can confirm the notice was taken over the telephone and the mistake was made whilst being typed up by the operator with your funeral director. Although this is a rare occurrence I agree that this is totally unacceptable and will ensure that the in-house trainers give any further support and training that may be required.

I can confirm the amendment was rectified for today's edition and I have now spoken with the funeral director this morning who will be contacting yourself today.

I would also like to take this opportunity to assure you and your family that we strive extremely hard to maintain our normal very high standard whilst placing bereavement notices and it is with great regret we didn't on this occasion. We and especially the operators do understand the impact such errors cause and it would never be our intention to cause families any further distress at what we know is an already sad and difficult time.

Kind regards

I then noted that in the bereavement section of the print edition of that same newspaper (January 9th 2017) the word 'inquiries' instead of 'enquiries' was used seven times in different death notices, which suggests that this was not a one-off mistake typed up by the operator over the telephone, but a longstanding systematic anomaly that has gone unchecked by successive editorial staff for years. I relayed this to senior staff at the publication and asked if any other relatives had complained about the misspelling. The very next day, on the 10th of January, the word 'inquiries' was erroneously appearing again in death notices on the bereavement page, which left me feeling very insulted that nothing was being done about this issue. I did a little more research and noticed that as far back as two months previous, the word 'inquiries' was mistakenly used for 'enquiries' in death notices. Astonishingly, I then checked another family member's death notice of November 2010 (seven years previous) and observed that the word 'inquiries' for 'enquiries' had been used then. After discussing it with other family members we were completely dumbfounded and found it unbelievable that this level of misspelling, over such a long period of time, could be commonplace and go unchecked.

I therefore concluded that if the newspaper were to compensate everybody with £100 for this anomaly (like they did me) it could run into hundreds of thousands of pounds.

Months later (July, 2018) the word 'inquiries' (instead of 'enquiries') appears to feature much less in the death notices.

Strange isn't it?

Diagnosing Doctor

Have you ever been to the doctor's surgery and the receptionist states something like, "I'll ask doctor" as though the doctor is the most important person in the world. This manner is designed to condition people that 'Doctor knows best' and we are just the mere mortal patients.

Doctor doesn't always know best. We are our own best doctors.

I have already detailed on many occasions the distress felt by patients forced to ask their GPs for support letters directly because our institutions demand that same evidence. Ordinary people are demeaned by the attitude of some doctors when asking for support, especially if it relates to benefits. This is in light of the fact that both government and CAB guidelines clearly state that applicants should contact their GP for letters of support.

Some GPs have refused point blank to put something in writing for patients (detailing illnesses/medical problems for example) by saying it is not in their remit. Whose remit is it in, then?

For example, if a patient is in need of a dosette box to monitor their medication, it has been reported that one doctor instructed the patient to obtain the letter from a chemist to prove they need special apparatus to monitor their drugs. DWP assessors clearly stipulate that they will only consider the use of a dosette box in making their decisions on disability if the evidence comes from the doctor.

On the contrary, doctors seem to be able to make such decisions when issuing sick notes and suchlike, but for benefits there is a stigma attached which is tantamount to discrimination.

Furthermore, if doctors do agree to write the patient a letter, many just want to regurgitate medical facts without making an opinion and/or they make sure they state, "The patient has asked me", or "The patient says". Doctors get paid a fee for this sort of ambiguous statement, may I add. In my experience, other doctors struggle to diagnose. Aren't doctors supposed to diagnose and to make statements as to what is their professional opinion? Maybe they are afraid that if they commit, they may be required to give further evidence under oath in a future lawsuit.

Some doctors are also reluctant to refer a patient to a specialist. One very assertive patient told how difficult he found it to secure a referral, which does not leave the non-assertive with much of a chance.

Would you believe that other doctors are completely ignorant of disabled issues and are most proficient at doling out antidepressants pushed by the massive pharmaceutical companies?

In conclusion, PIP (Personal Independence Payment) and ESA (Employment Support Allowance) application/assessments can be a seriously distressing time for the vulnerable and those with mental health problems – in fact some commit suicide directly because of it.

Doctors are not helping matters.

The IRA Didn't Win the War, Sinn Fein Did

It seems an odd statement to make, that IRA violence worked. In spite of this, James Prior (now Baron Prior) the Northern Ireland Secretary who served under Margaret Thatcher, said just that in a BBC documentary *Who Won The War?* (broadcast in October 2014).

By contrast, could we ask the same question, as in, did British violence committed in Ireland over the years work?

Apparently, violence perpetrated by the British to settle the Irish Question has for centuries been indicative of their bullyboy warring mindset. From Cromwell putting two thousand to the sword in Drogheda in 1649, the Oath of Supremacy blackmail, the Black and Tans' persecution of the Irish populace after 1920, to Bloody Sunday 1972, it has been never-ending.

Then there were those subtle massacres like that of the potato famine of 1848 (otherwise known as Britain's holocaust).

Getting back to the question, the answer is yes, British-sponsored violence in Eire (both north and south) has worked since time immemorial.

With regard to the bold statement of who won the war, in relation to the ceasefires of 1994 and 1996 one could argue that British unionism won, being cognisant that the UK status quo remains.

Yet this does not take into account the massive gains Sinn Fein has made in the twenty-six counties (known as the Republic of Ireland) where it now holds 15% of the vote (and growing) and has secured a record number of local councillors. This is in contrast, of course, to the 1990s, when the Irish nationalist party barely held 1% of the vote.

This is coupled with the fact that Sinn Fein are currently not just in government but are the largest party in Northern Ireland (the expropriated six counties).

Others might argue that the key to unlocking both a geographical and political change (a united Ireland) lies in Sinn Fein forming a government in southern Ireland whereas all-Ireland institutions can begin to facilitate that independence.

Unlike their British counterparts (who during the recent troubles of 1969–1996 subjugated and coerced dissenting Catholics in the north by threat and terror) it is believed that nationalists are to use the power of persuasion in relation to the Protestant minority on the island. This could be initiated by affecting compelling cross-border institutions (like health and employment) whereby both Catholics and Protestants can be inclusive (most Catholics in Northern Ireland already hold an Irish passport).

Regarding the issue of who won the war; there are no victors in war, only losers. Is it not the ordinary people of Ireland and Britain who have won out, now that sectarian brutality (like the Shankill butchery) and civilian atrocities like Enniskillen and Birmingham (after which hatred mutated into a deeper variant) has ceased?

By the same token, the BBC documentary to mark the 20th anniversary of the IRA and loyalist ceasefires of 1994 is a little misplaced, taking into account that after the IRA cessation of 1994 there was the Docklands bombing (Canary Wharf). Conclusively, the IRA detonated a device in London's financial district in 1996 which was to be the defining moment in the conflict (some even describing it as a military masterstroke).

Remembering that the Bishopsgate bombing of 1993 (Bishopsgate being the main thoroughfare in London's financial district) had already caused rumours to circulate that the massive financial organisations in London were considering relocating to Frankfurt.

Therefore the sceptics would assert that it was financial loss, not civilian loss, that was the reason the British negotiated over Ireland; taking into consideration the British Prime Minister of the time John Major's prolonged and histrionic insistence that there must be words like 'permanent' inscribed in any Provisional armistice.

One should also not forget the daring rocket attack on 10 Downing Street that pre-dated the bomb blasts of 1993 and 1996. In February 1991 there was an attempt to assassinate the British war cabinet, meeting to discuss the Gulf War.

Concurrently, festering in the British political psyche, would be the 1984 bombing of the Grand Hotel in Brighton when the ruling Conservative government was nearly wiped out. In that very hotel, IRA volunteer Patrick Magee had the temerity to book a room and plant a device that would bring mayhem to the established elite attending a Tory Party conference. Over three weeks before the event Magee had checked into the hotel under the fictitious name of Roy Walsh to prime a 20–30lb bomb hidden in a bathroom wall.

Love's a Disease

I can never forget a story read in my local newspaper some years back. It was concerning a dispute between two young women vying for the affection of one young man. Anyway, to cut a long story short, the consequences were that outside the Out of Town inn on Town Road, Hanley, and in a fit of jealous rage, one young woman pulled the other's skirt right down to her ankles. This set me thinking as to what love is and how it renders us. Some believe it is a basic chemical reaction between one person and another, where the heart wavers, the stomach flips over, and one becomes obsessed by the other where it can be equal and fulfilling.

This was epitomised more recently (August 2017) while on the tube at London Bridge. A youngish-looking couple opposite appeared trance-like in their apparent 'love' for each other. Yes, it was so sickly-grin time it would send the most romantic amongst us running for the sick bucket; especially when the female rubbed suntan cream in the male's face, all the time staring starry-eyed at one another, both lost in that dreamy daze.

Opposingly, for some it's not all strawberries and cream (or suntan lotion). Am I identifying a new species when describing that the love obsession can be all-consuming, gradually at first, just like the Lust Worm burrowing into the brain. When fully engorged that worm can then disable, it can confuse and it can be so intense, those under its influence can actually kill themselves or others because of it, sometimes because 'they couldn't live without them'. Some of those in love also don't eat or sleep because the phenomenon governs their entire thought processes, by and large centred on the over-analysis of simple innocent comments the partner may utter. As in when they do manage to fall sleep (unconsciousness being the only respite) the object of their desire is the last face they see. Not to mention that the first seconds of brain function in the waking hour centres on that one same person again. Talk about debilitating.

Many in the love state cannot hold a conversation with an outside party unless they are associating a simple topic (like the weather) as a comparison as to whether their loved one would hold that same view. What's more, such is the degree of wanting to control another when being bitten by the love bug one can play mind games with their loved one in pertaining to be super popular to relay the message that they will always be desired elsewhere in the event of possible rejection. But why do we seek out this 'love' state of being and why does it determine our lives? Reproductive programming could be the answer to this conundrum as in the genetic need to procreate and pair up with a mate overrides anything else. It is not dissimilar to our requirement for food, shelter and security, which begs the question: how many couples are involved and committed to unloving relationships because they are terrified to be alone?

This brings into the equation the double dichotomy of: can two people love each other with the same velocity, and can you truly grow to love somebody in the context of a relationship? Furthermore, can that growing love be just as powerful as the 'love at first sight' variety? After all, many desire passion as a pre-requisite to a loving relationship, don't they?

It also goes without saying that invariably, one partner loves the other either more, or less, than the other partner. Is it therefore better to love a partner less and always wonder what one is missing, or is it better to love your mate more and experience all the torment that inevitably fits that descriptor?

Conclusively, if one's love is on the tepid side would one be less hurt if the relationship should end? After all, the realist would say the average relationship only lasts for seven years in any event. If the love does not break down naturally over time, death will inevitably bring about its demise. This in turn, brings about the question as to what happens when love dies a natural death. As in one partner just does not love the other anymore? Is it comparable to a dispossession as in one should not curl up and die in distress but breathe a sigh of relief? After all, that haunted look after riding the roller coaster of emotions was not exactly fun, was it?

Was it Wilde or Tennyson who said: "Better to have loved and lost than never to have loved at all"?

Hmm; not convinced on that one.

Middleport Pottery –
A Time Capsule of its Own

Time capsules don't necessarily have to be buried for future generations to unearth; they can be restored and put on display to educate the present.

The Middleport Pottery Visitor Centre in Port Street, Burslem, has been restored and exhibited for the whole world to see, and as far as Victorian authenticity goes, it is indeed world class. Furthermore, the tissue transfer technique, perfected by Josiah Spode in 1784 and used throughout the era, is done in exactly the same fashion today.

The Prince's Regeneration Trust invested £9 million on revamping the works, which has produced Burleigh china since 1888. Moreover, it is the only Victorian pottery factory that is still operational.

I have always been fascinated by the arbitrary Victorian model (especially local), including the priggish and puritanical upper, middle and lower class sociology.

In fact I am drawn to that age like a moth to a flame.

On entrance to Middleport Pottery, the first sense to be exercised is that of smell, you know, that old nostalgic odour that accompanies the more passé constructions. The interior offices strike you to imagine that in escaping the outside world to enter Middleport Pottery, you have vacated a real-life time machine and one was now most definitely immersed in the past.

If you do visit and the antique black telephone rings, pick it up and put on your best telephone voice – it could be a royal connection. I answered it and no, for doing so I didn't get scolded by a strait-laced governess.

It was when moving upstairs on the site that I was to sensate the most atmospheric stimulation that I had ever experienced whilst visiting any other like attraction (even the Dickens Museum in London). The sensation was so unusual, I exited the room and re-entered to encounter it again. That same area led to another chamber which permeated that same mysterious ambiance.

It was most delightful to eat your lunch at the canal side. Bumblebees in striped fur coats flitted from flower to flower nearby. Barges also chugged along the waterway to illustrate the serene picturesque summer setting (August 2018) against the backdrop of stern industrial Victorianism.

I had discerned fox droppings on the yard beside the canal and imagined how local workers reacted to foxes in that aeon. Surely there was barely enough food for the workers, never mind the sly old fox? Perhaps the foxes ate the rats and mice, I contemplated.

And perhaps the pottery workers ate morsels of dry bread and dripping.

At the canal side, I could see the crane that loaded the exports onto barges in the 19th Century and I tried to visualise other, more moving, sequences. Would hands already be cut from handling the sharp biscuit ware, as heavy crates were loaded? Would thick smog be billowing from all seven bottle ovens? In addition, was shovelling coal to keep the kilns fired at night a prized post, in mind that it would keep one warm on a cold winter's night?

It was at this point that I cast my mind back to the early 1970s, when we used to walk along the canal route from Hanley, via Etruria, to Westport Lake. I can vaguely remember many used, disused and derelict foundries along the way.

Middleport Pottery must have been one of them.

I could recall finding a baby grebe before it was lost and putting it into a disused train truck where we thought our newfound pet would be safe. As a ten-year-old I was shocked to discover on returning the next day that the bird had perished and was crawling with ants.

I then looked over to the other side of the canal (presently) and wished that just for one moment, I could see my friends and myself walking along that path, all those years ago.

What would we be wearing and what would we be talking about?

Yes, that is why time machines, time capsules, time travel and anything to do with the passage of time have always been so captivating to humankind.

Middleport Pottery most certainly transports the visitor back to that time.

Do Judge a Book by its Cover

During a legal battle with my social landlord some years ago, where many faults including fire issues were brought to notice, the response not just from the landlord but from the fire service and other related institutions (including legal institutions) was disgraceful.

A site visit by a judge had been initiated, so that the judge could inspect the flats complex relating to the court case. The complaints included stair grips (or nosings) that were working loose, and dangerous outside concrete slab trip hazards, to name just two issues.

I had also received a court order stating that another person could not support me during the judge's visit. This was discussed on the telephone with a court adviser who categorically stated that nobody could accompany me for the visit. Later, the CAB advised that by law, I could have a McKenzie friend to accompany me for moral support. So the advice given by the court, together with the court order, were inappropriate, to say the least. It seems that the usual utterance from many court officials when I have visited is 'we cannot give legal advice' but as proved by the misleading court order and the bad advice given by the court official; they can give legal mis-advice.

As my supporter and I waited for the judge to arrive, it was alarming to see three people walk into the complex. They comprised a member of the legal defence team, a representative of the social landlord (the defendant) and the judge. When the judge introduced himself I explained the reasons behind the McKenzie friend and asked the judge how come two people were present for the defence when the court order had clearly stipulated that there should only be one? Furthermore, I asked how come the two representatives for the defence were accompanying the judge entering the flats complex when he was supposed to be independent? This was not compatible with my right to a fair hearing.

How would it have looked if I had walked into the complex in a familiar manner arm in arm with the judge, taking into consideration that he was supposed to be neutral? On top of that, where did the judge meet up with the defence and on whose orders?

When it was pointed out to the judge that I had been told not to bring anybody for support during the visit, he mumbled something about not wanting many people present (or something along those lines). Perish the thought of the even greater manipulation and intimidation I would have felt had I not brought along a supporter.

In reference to the judge, it seemed he had a set agenda. He could not reason with me regarding the hazards but looked to find nothing wrong at the complex. After showing him a dangerous, loose paving stone at the front of the complex he dismissed it because it was not in the court order; even though I mentioned that a loose slab was dangerous whether at the front or rear of the complex. When I later pinpointed a loose slab at the rear exit and pointed out the design fault of the concrete he said, "Where is the trip hazard, Mr. Raftery?" It was plain for all to see where the trip hazard was and so I became suspicious of his reasoning. I therefore said to my supporter, "Can you see a trip hazard?" To which they replied, "It's obvious there is a trip hazard," at which the judge started to make notes. I then asked the judge to come and look at the hazardous concrete area (which another judge at another hearing had already called 'crude concrete which offends building regulations') from a different angle, which he reluctantly did.

In fact, the loose slabs in question had been a hazard for months. Over those months different witnesses had seen this hazard and still it was not made safe under the landlord's repairing obligations. One of the witnesses to these hazards was a housing standards officer from the council.

Regarding the stair grips being loose, the judge had asked if the grips were all right at this time, to which I replied they seemed to be okay on that day. It can be argued that since the initial case and the subsequent injunction attempt against the social landlord the grips problem had been addressed and made safer for all the residents, although I, and many others, had suffered for years because the landlord had consistently refused to repair them.

There was also documentary evidence from the housing provider that the screws holding the stair grips in place still worked loose from time to time. Regardless, the judge's reasoning was that because none were loose on that day there was no fault to report. The same could be said for the other matter to be investigated during the site visit (the new storage heater) in that since the injunction application I had been fitted with a new heater (and even that one had caused disastrous problems including damp smoke). To conclude the visit, the judge and the defence team representative started to discuss the case in legal terms as if it were the defence team taking the case. I reminded them there and then that it was my case and it was not being manipulated by the defence to suit; just because they had legal expertise.

After just a few days I noticed that the loose slab had been 'crudely' stuck down or something like, in attempt to make it safe.

Blonde Bombshells of 1943: A Review

I am not what one would call a theatre buff; but have to say the playhouse is a welcoming break from the cinema. Perhaps I was spoilt when I saw the brilliant *Chitty Chitty Bang Bang* at the London Palladium some years back. The songs were excellent. Then again, *Evita,* when seen at the Regent in Hanley, was not enjoyed as much because it was a sung-through (no dialogue at all). I also viewed the highbrow *Swan Lake* in Prague and while waiting for curtain up, could not help but imagine a play within a play starring the Elephant Man seated in Baroness Burdett-Coutts' private box, marvelling at the theatrics.

Anyhow, you can take the man out of Stoke but you can't take Stoke out of the man, so they say. When a ballerina on stage fairied around in her flowing white gown, I was compelled to shout:

"You've still got yer nighty on duck."

Costing £12 at the New Vic Theatre in Basford in 2013, *Blonde Bombshells of 1943* by Alan Plater is not everybody's cup of tea. In saying that, the musical-cum-comedy sketches, set in Northern England during wartime, did deem it an unusual act to follow.

Many, it appeared, enjoyed this particular cup of tea because the New Vic was packed to the rafters by a predominantly older audience who chuckled away at the puerile one-liners from the seven women on stage; for example, one of the *Bombshell* actresses stated that she thought Lesbians was the capital of Portugal.

Being sceptical myself and not amused by the gags, it was pointed out that this silly type of joke was commonplace during that era and the actors on stage were portraying this accurately.

Perhaps the jury might be out on that one.

Having a predilection for harsh/dark Dickensian plots I gave the show a chance, and after sitting through line after line of what I deemed unfunny jokes (mainly accentuated by the typically blunt and brassy Grace, played by Natasha White) the show seemed to perhaps improve when the only male member of the crew made his entrance, auditioning as a drummer for the all-girl band (at this point I was beginning to wonder whether anyone would notice if I waited in the theatre bar until the show was over).

The 'script' then saw the young and handsome conscription evader, 'Patrick' (Chris Grahamson), join the musical grouping, thus evading detection from the war authorities by donning a pink dress and blonde wig. This saw an unusual transvestite twist to the theatrical proceedings.

On the plus side, the musical skill of the women (and the man) playing the instruments was of a high level and some of the songs from the Swing period were nostalgic, to say the least. At one interval during the show, I wondered how the actors managed the circular set and kept imagining the front stage scenario, in that perhaps I was missing something when the company had to turn around to face other sections of the audience.

Danielle Potts, 25, of Clayton, who was in the audience, most definitely believed it was her cup of Rosy Lee. She said, post show:

"It was a good laugh, but it would have been more entertaining if more soldiers had been in the show; I don't know if I found Patrick, the lead male character, good-looking or not. My cast favourite was Grace, who was down to earth and cracked some good jokes. As far as the music is concerned it is not the music I would normally listen to, but I did enjoy it because it accompanied the war years."

Imprinted

I first ran for council in the local elections on May 5th 2014 and, as a novice, was ignorant of the prerequisite regarding imprints on leaflets. In that same year, I was informed verbally (nothing came in writing) that someone had reported the fact that the appropriate name and address (imprint) was not on my leaflets. As such, I included the imprint on the next batch of leaflets.

In the local elections of May 5th 2016, I decided to run with a party who, I discovered at the last minute, had left me 500 leaflets short. As a result, I hastily decided to make some up for myself. There was not much time left and I started to become anxious (there is email evidence between the party and me regarding this unforeseen circumstance).

I then rushed the leaflet in designing it (this was relayed to my contact at the printers). I do remember asking the contact to put the name and address at the bottom of the leaflet. I cannot remember anything else.

Therefore, I did not knowingly omit the full imprint (the printer's name was on the leaflet, my name and address was not) and did not intend to defraud anyone by forgetting to add the full imprint. In reality, forgetting to include my name and address on the imprint was something I had no control over.

Then, on Friday 6th May 2016, I received a threatening email from a DC of the Major Organised Crime Team, Fraud and Financial Investigations Unit. Thereafter, I was terrified and distressed all over the weekend. In effect, it was unfair to have this matter hanging over me that same weekend. On the Friday, I had tried to call the DC a few times but was asked by a recording to submit a pin number. Besides, for a detective to become involved because I had inadvertently left my name and/or address off a leaflet was a disproportionate response to the alleged offence. As in, why was this not a matter for the council or the Electoral Commission? I contacted the Electoral Commission myself and relayed the story. As a result, I was mystified as to where they recruit staff members and how those staff are trained, such was their toothless desperation to side with the council.

Fraud definition

Wrongful or criminal deception intended to result in financial or personal gain.

In fact, the email from the DC implied that I was suspected of being a major organised criminal – for leaving words off a leaflet.

I then wrote to the DC in question via email to explain the situation and the mitigating circumstances and received a voicemail message on Monday 9th May 2016 from him, in which he apologised for any distress caused and also said that he was not going to pursue the matter. On calling him back, he categorically stated that the new returning officer at the council had reported the matter to him and had not mentioned any mitigating circumstances. Shockingly, two conflicting versions of events then arose.

The DC clearly and concisely informed me over the telephone that another candidate had reported the imprint offence to the then current returning officer at the council, who had then, in turn, reported it to the police. The police officer would not disclose which candidate reported the 'offence'. Conflictingly, when questioned, the returning officer categorically stated via email that a member of the public had reported the offence. He said that:

"I can confirm that an elector for the Town ward passed a copy of the leaflet to me last Tuesday, 3rd May. The complaint and the leaflet were passed to the police single-point-of-contact as the returning officer is obliged to do under guidance from the Electoral Commission.

As this is now being investigated by the police, I cannot comment further."

As any reasonable person can deduce, there are two versions of events from two different public figures.

It is therefore believed that the returning officer should have made enquiries regarding any mitigating circumstance before he reported to the police. His colleagues were also aware of the background to the case because they were the subject of an Ombudsman investigation in 2014 because one of them had made inappropriate comments about memory. I have email evidence that several council employees (mainly from elections) all knew about the mitigating factors.

*Reporting allegations of electoral fraud 1.53: If you are concerned that electoral fraud may have been committed, you should first speak to the Electoral Registration Officer or the Returning Officer. 1.54: They may be able to explain whether or not electoral fraud has been committed, and can refer your concerns to the police **if necessary**. They can also provide you with the details of the police contact for the relevant police force so that you can report the allegation yourself.*

It is fair to say that although it is recognised that the police were following procedure and could not have known about the mitigating circumstance surrounding the 'imprint offence', their response was disproportionate to the offence alleged. Even though I had forgotten to include my name and address on a leaflet, my full name and credentials were all over that said leaflet. The initial email from the DC was threatening and I felt harassed by it.

What's more, the police now have me registered where a record of the allegation is to be retained at the Fraud Unit under reference 357.16. I have not committed fraud or attempted to commit fraud.

I feel that a simple telephone call from the investigating police officer regarding the imprint matter would have resulted in him learning about the build-up to the 'offence' and the unforeseen circumstances surrounding the imprint omission, without the need to terrorise me with the email. In reality, the course of action pursued by the DC could be construed as professional misconduct or something more serious, like harassment.

It must be said that when I first omitted the imprint because of inexperience in 2014, the returning officer of the time did not report it or document it. Back in 2014, I received a telephone call from that same returning officer to advise that the imprint had been omitted and so I immediately addressed the matter.

This time around the new returning officer did not make any enquiries amongst the elections team regarding possible previous incidents and so was not made aware of the first imprint matter with the first returning officer two years earlier. The point being that if it is protocol to report to the police every time there is an imprint offence, the returning officer two years ago should have reported it.

Therefore, the argument that the imprint was reported to the police because it was my second offence is not credible.

After putting in a complaint to both the council and the police, the police were the more transparent.

In paragraph six of the letter from the investigating police representative dated 16th June 2015, it is clearly stated that the council did know of my mitigating circumstances and they failed to share pertinent information to the police. The investigating officer then went on to say that in future cases, he would make sure that the question would be asked if there were any mitigating factors to be aware of, making sure the police were sensitive to the needs of the individual.

Amusements to be had in Sunny Rhyl

Nineteen seventy-five, when I was a twelve-year-old having moved from Stoke-on-Trent to Kinmel Bay near Rhyl, North Wales with my family, saw me running back to Stoke every time there was an argument, usually with no money in my pocket and nowhere to stay. After a few months and being caught repeatedly at Crewe railway station without a ticket, I began to settle down and realised Rhyl had more to it than the, by now, exhausted beach.

I attended Blessed Edward Jones High School on Cefndy Road and soon realised that 'fiddling' was the name of the game and the amusement arcades offered much more than amusement. Yet, perhaps it helped that I had always been cheeky hard-faced; when using our bus pass out of school hours, others would hold their pass out for a long time for the bus driver to examine, only for the driver to realise it was invalid at that hour and so would not let them on to the bus. I, on the other hand, would whizz past the driver like lightning, flashing the pass for a split second viewing so the driver did not have time to scrutinise it. I would then head straight to the back seat of the bus where I would usually light up. I was definitely not the diffident type; as a twelve-, thirteen- and fourteen-year-old nothing or no one seemed to faze me.

It was then cursorily deduced that one didn't put money into the slot machines; one took money out. It began with waiting for the pennies to fall from the penny pusher due to a lucky vibration, to banging the machines to make the pennies drop, to inserting paper clips into the slots of the wheel-em-in, to the five and the one trick, then advancing to the Yale lock master key

64

scenario which opened up the cash boxes to the kiddies' rides. The arcades recalled are the Carousel, Pleasureland, The Brightspot and Sands Arcade (the latter of which can be seen in the 1973 film, *Holiday on the Buses*).

Banging the machines had inevitably escalated to lifting them up and dropping them down, so the pennies would fall over the edge of that little cliff inside the machine. The Flipper Winner penny pusher saw piles of pennies on two levels and when undertaking the lift and drop mechanism the pennies just cascaded down into the tray below, but you had to make a quick getaway, which was doable because the machine was right next to the entrance/exit and was not alarmed.

The wheel-em-in stunt (where you had to roll the penny down the slot to fit it in between those lines in order to win) was the most curious. We would buy paper clips and open them out into the letter S. Then we would insert one into the slot of the wheel-em-in, where you were supposed to put your penny, blow down the slot and the paper clip would then be seen inside the machine on the moving circuit. Oddly enough, when the paper clip got to the end of that circuit and disappeared over the edge out of sight, the money would keep gushing out from the top of the machine and roll down the glass into my eager outstretched hands. I don't know why this happened; I just gleefully mopped up the loot in unison to the clicking sound of the coppers being pumped out.

The five and the one trick was when you put a 5p piece into the change slot and a 1p piece in the standard slot of a one-armed-bandit at the same time; you then pulled the arm lever as if to play, at the same time, and for some strange reason, pennies dropped out.

The best way to get rid of your newly-accrued wealth, which was by now weighing down your pockets, was to walk up and down Rhyl promenade asking holidaymakers, "Have you got a ten pence piece, please?" to which you would dump ten penny pieces on them. I don't recall anyone ever complaining about being dumped on.

Then there was bingo, where we would 'play in the dark' (without putting the 5p into the slot to light up the board) and if you won, you would put your 5p in and shout house at the same time to muffle out the sound of the coin dropping in to light up the board. Another ruse was that if we knew the bingo checker from school, they would shout out false numbers when checking a bogie call, one school friend was also a bingo caller and would call out our numbers.

If you were clocked by an attendant (sometimes in grey overalls) on the fiddle in the amusement arcades the local saying was 'knicks'. A school friend rasped this expression when on a fiddling expedition with an acquaintance who had possession of the master key. This Yale lock key opened most of the cash boxes fitted with Yale locks on children's rides that cost 5p or 10p. After splitting up, as a result of calling a false knicks (while holding the key) he swiftly got the key cut and then of course I got a cut of the key too.

We had struck arcade gold and had advanced into the big time.

Not content with emptying the cashboxes in the Rhyl area, we went out as far as Abergele, Talacre and even Blackpool, but our speciality was a children's ride called Pongo on the main road in Towyn. In the winter months when there were no holidaymakers to fill up the cash boxes, we would often laugh and scrap for Pongo's last 5p.

Yes, I have fond memories of my mate Pongo even when times were hard.

No doubt all good things come to an end, and as a sixteen-year-old I was rumbled just inside an arcade next to the Brightspot. I used to hide my key in the waistband of my trousers and after I tried the lion ride outside the arcade (you had to see if the key would open it) an attendant became suspicious and brought me inside to search me. As I then walked out, a little chime was audible as my key hit the deck. I did not dare to turn around and acknowledge it. So that was that.

After leaving Blessed Edward Jones in 1978, some would argue I had obtained not just a good state education but had also graduated via the *Free School of Machine Coinage* and had gained the equivalent of a First in Arcade Culture (both theory and practice). Although Carol Vorderman was also a pupil at Blessed Edward Jones High School and went on to attain a third class degree in Engineering at Cambridge University, I can't imagine her having to perfect her mathematical enumeration by counting (the lack of) 5p pieces in Pongo's cash box – can you?

The Chairman and the Editor

Personally speaking; the story regarding the Port Vale chairman's ban on our local paper from entering the press box in 2013 was the most intriguing local story for years.

Due to the fact that there has been a swift moratorium of civilities between the two parties, it did not take a football genius to work out what went wrong in allowing the standoff to occur. More remarkable was the newspaper editor's response to the situation. In his heartfelt plea to the Port Vale chairman, Norman Smurthwaite, he mentioned his first name (Norman) seventeen times in the piece.

Talk about labouring the point.

Then, to get Port Vale fans on side, the editor attempted to court favour from the dinosaur 'National Sports Writers' who hold no sway with ordinary Vale fans one can safely argue.

The statement published in the local newspaper regarding the chairman said that, "he has attended three awards ceremonies as a guest of the Sentinel, and never paid a penny," also defied belief.

In his club statement and in the build-up to the banning, the Port Vale chairman said he befriended a member of the local paper's team and had passed on information to him, who in turn, then divulged that confidential information to the sports editor of that same paper.

Local newspapers and chairmen/staff of football clubs should not be disclosing information to each other of any description, and by all accounts they should establish a professional relationship and a professional relationship only. In fact, these cohorts should not be inviting each other to fancy functions and disclosing club (or some would say public) information along the way, period.

Local newspapers should not think they are infallible because they provide the club with free advertisement/projection. It could be surprising just how quickly supporters could get used to their club not featuring in the local press.

In saying that, those who are not conversant with the Internet would suffer as a result of this kind of dispute the longer it went on.

It was doubly interesting when the editor paraphrased the chairman in his 'heartfelt plea' to the Vale fans. In doing so he exemplified the problem:

"It's interesting that his tweets state: 'no more freebies... end of' and 'no more free lunches'" in reference to us.

There should be no free lunches full stop.

The moral to this low, bickering-themed story is that those who have the means to pay are given an exemption not to pay – whereas those on a low income like ordinary fans are consistently stung. Where is the logic in that?

The over-friendly relationship between the local paper and Port Vale would need to become a thing of the past if both parties want to resume some kind of semblance of normality in the future.

And as for the newspaper reporters not being allowed in the cushy Port Vale press box; they should have done what I and others have had to do when writing on/supporting Port Vale... pay your entrance fee and rough it.

Galapagos:
Islands that Time Forgot

Those once-in-a-lifetime experiences are entitled such because we only do them once. When we do visit obscure and renowned places (like the Galapagos Islands off the South American country of Ecuador) what can be just as provocative is to recognise the slow unmoving mess we have left behind. There is no better insight than to leave your own insular hamster's wheel and propel yourself to the outside looking in. The Galapagos Islands slice of the unknown affords one that privilege.

I had to Google what an archipelago is, and for the record, it appears to be geographical jargon for a cluster of islands. The word archipelago seemed to be liberally banded around Santa Cruz (perhaps the most central island of the Galapagos chain situated in the middle of the Pacific Ocean straddling the equator) especially at the Charles Darwin Research Centre in town.

To begin, perhaps it is best to mull over the theory of how the big ape (airline passengers in this case) cannot stow laptops or other valuables in the hold in case they go missing. How can this be so with safety supposed to be so overriding at all airports? If your laptop could go 'walkies' the airline must be employing untrustworthy personnel, which is a security risk. Not content with lugging a heavy laptop and cumbersome charger around, I brought along an iPad instead and paid the price when writing up the skeletal frame for this piece. It was exasperating, singularly bonging on those keys like a primitive baboon.

On my very first day, when bearing witness (from behind the police checkpoint) to the statuesque marine iguana extraordinaire, all grouped and frozen still on a rock, it was quickly deduced that dinosaurs did not become extinct, they modified, became smaller and eventually became us. This idea was cemented when sighting the giant tortoise on an expedition to the highlands of Santa Cruz. Not over-enthused with these slow-moving creatures, the giant tortoise bestowed on the encounter an almost science fiction or 'Land of the Giants' scenario. How fascinating that this reptile can live up to 200 years old, which would make it a modern-day dinosaur in itself.

It is without question that we evolved from sea creatures like the iguana. Not only has our skin layering system developed accordingly, due to millions of years of battles with nature, we have a propensity to many more human-reptilian characteristics if we were to examine ourselves more closely.

The frigates flying overhead on Santa Cruz also reminded one of a back to front Tyrannosaurus Rex. And those peculiar pelicans – what characters. These odd creatures wait patiently, staring at the fishmonger, hopefully awaiting a morsel, with pleading expressions. They then all lurch their bodies forward slightly, in unison, if they detect that a fishy titbit might be coming their way. The finale being an all-squawking comical flapping scrummage when that fishy carrion is eventually thrown to the eager, feathered ensemble. What a spectacle. It's another surreal dimension beyond; never mind the dinosaur.

Staying tuned to the dinosaur theme, it was on a half-day trip to Las Greitas on Santa Cruz with an accompanying chaperone that our hypocrisy regarding other species was reinforced.

After witnessing a very special moment when a cactus finch went about its daily cacti manoeuvres right in front of my watching eyes, I was informed that a heron (pointed out near to the pink salt marshes) only ate baby iguanas. It was therefore pondered that if the scheme of things were different, how horrified we would be if there existed a large dinosaur-like beast who only had a fancy to lunch on human babies. Is it therefore only by chance that we are in pole position with regard to the food chain strata? In this situation, and as human beings, we would have had to adapt to the abhorrent circumstance of our babies being prey, wouldn't we? Just like sheep have adapted to us taking their babies (lambs) away and eating them.

When visiting the Charles Darwin Research Centre in Puerto Ayora, it was discovered that our most eminent scientist landed his ship (the Beagle) at San Cristobel (another Galapagos island) in 1835. Therein, Darwin's crew helped decimate the giant tortoise indigenous to the islands; yes, they ate them. It must also be said that the Charles Darwin Research Centre was a very interesting place to hang out (the lovely cool air conditioning was also a big plus). For a change, I found the patience to read every noticeboard to enlighten myself with the facts and pondered if those nasty, big red-eyed bluebottles (*Philornis downsi)* that attack and harm the young mangrove finch are the same ones which terrorise swimmers on the beach, apparently attracted to the salt water bodily encrusted. If this is the case, I would gladly hunt them down to extinction myself.

Some could argue that researchers at the Centre are still atoning for the tortoise slaughter. In reference to the current research, one can't help but imagine that although great work is being undertaken, the researchers could be interfering too. This can be seen by the losing battle being waged against the invasive blackberry on Galapagos and the introduction of the ladybird/ moth to restore or protect native plant life. This is in direct contradiction to Darwin's theories, which is espoused all over the islands, in that all living things must adapt or die (which includes the giant tortoise). Darwin also argued that it's not the most intelligent or the strongest/fittest who survive, but those most adaptable. Surely though, the creatures (including us) with inclined intelligence would be those who would be most aware that they must adjust to outlast. Our Charlie wasn't always theory-perfect you know, and as stated in other pieces, his privileged background would be to his overall detriment in some ways. In making this point, if Darwin had not been conceived from a privileged background, he would not have had the means to make the voyage to the Galapagos Islands in the first place and would be as renowned today as an East End barrow boy. Now let's see, keeping with Darwinian theory, the next paragraph highlights natural evolutionary ideas, but in more depth. Even so, it must be said that all opinion is subjective by design and this is another such view among the glutted environmental/ evolutionary voices out there.

Nobody disputes that the finch migrated to the Galapagos Islands millions of years ago and more than likely brought with it lice (pest). Man arrived more recently and brought with him rodents, goats and cats (pest) and decimated the tortoise population simultaneously. If man had not brought the invader, floating masses of vegetation or land breaks could have introduced those same species to the islands. Therefore, we do not know how the Galapagos Islands were meant to evolve if man has interfered in controlling the numbers of invasive species as seen today. For example, would the iguana have retreated into the ocean permanently in order to survive once it realised it would have to adapt to new predators (like wild cats) on land? More bizarre still, could the iguana, over millions of years of evolution, develop wings to escape predation?

Are we therefore hampering the natural course of events?

Regarding the giant tortoise and the wider argument, it is thought goats must be controlled because they feed on grass meant for the tortoise. But what if man is not here in the future to bail the reptile out; how will the tortoise survive if they do not learn the skills themselves? The idea propagated that animal life on the islands is not used to predators so show no fear towards them is a nonsense. They will soon learn and adjust, just like the crabs have done when approached by humans – they scarper for cover under the rocks.

To expand a little, the finch should be brought into the equation to demonstrate the unhealthy affect human beings are having on animal life on the Galapagos Islands (vehicle pollution is stating the obvious). At breakfast time at the hotel (breakfast consisting of stale buns put into the oven to soften them up), I declined to eat with the other guests and much preferred dining with the finches. After all, who wants to bear witness to the human cement mixer machinations first thing. It was such a delight when multiple species of finch hovered around for a morsel. Even so, I could not help but observe that they were feeding on our unhealthy tourist diet of white bread, cheap margarine and cheap jams, and this was occurring at every hotel all over the islands. This diet over a long period could pose serious health problems for the finch, including stunted growth and a narrowing of the arteries. We can still dine with the finch by being provided with nuts and seeds for our porridge – a simple and inexpensive solution.

On a psychological note, another poser manifested itself when a knowledgeable tour guide disclosed that only the male iguana dives into the sea to forage for food (the female stays put). We know that same-sex relationships happen in the animal kingdom, so what would occur if two female iguanas set up nest? Would one assume the male role and forage into the sea or would they both assume the female role and maybe starve to death by staying put? The notion of whether other animals purposely psychologically abuse/reject/neglect their young, like human beings do, also occurred. Yes, many would concur that a visit to the Galapagos is not akin to a holiday but a thought-provoking research experience. Staying with animal psychology, I posed the idea to the 'diver types' at the hotel who had visited the world-renowned Gordon Rocks to dive with sharks and sunfish, that sooner or later one of those 'docile' sharks was going to suffer from a mental health problem and go for them. It was also suggested that an uninvited rogue great white could turn up to the diving party. I had seen the great white in action tearing into rotten flesh off the coast of Cape Town; not to be trifled with. Perhaps I was a tad jealous because I was not donning a wet suit – who knows?

It has to be said that one quickly accepts that to tour the Galapagos Islands the visitor must travel and pay (there is a $100-dollar entrance fee to the islands). Supermarket prices are also exceptionally high. Most trips out to see the animals are around the £100 mark and include snorkelling as the only means of discovery. My first excursion in one of those fast passenger speed-boats (to the island of Isabela) took two hours there and two hours back and would best be described as 'arduous' (but for the entertaining motley crew of half-drunk English and Canadians). The second trip to Floreana took approximately the same amount of time and could be deemed as laborious, with the third trip, to Pinzon, best summed up as 'gruelling'. Nonetheless, it was all well worth it. At Isabela it was observed how territorial the sea lions (or fur seals – both are indigenous to the Galapagos) had become; they had the run of the place. The seals were in fact splayed out over public benches and when I lightly touched one on the back (I am one of those naughty types who doesn't always listen to orders), the seal emanated a sort of muted yelp and lunged at me, shuffling over in my direction. In response, I mutedly yelped too, instantaneously bolting the vicinity. A sea lion had already growled at me from the seashore to let me know who was in charge. As far as I was concerned, those displayed fish-tearing teeth could have taken my hand off and I was taking no chances.

One of those very slightly aggressive seals could have been the same creature I saw awkwardly hauling its blubber over the sand minutes earlier, pooing as it clumsily bungled its way along. Yes, we're not all big fans of those cuddly, seemingly smiling, furry seals. In fact, I was dismayed there was no insect expedition at Isabela, as seen in the Amazon rainforest, when we were introduced to the soldier ants. (I did unearth a strange moth on a window ledge on Santa Cruz which had an identical tail fin to that of an aircraft. I declared that I had discovered a new species conducive to advanced aerodynamics).

In fact, I much preferred sunbathing with the black iguanas, who seemed to enjoy just lying there soaking up the rays. And yes, I committed the immortal Galapagos sin once again; with some spontaneity, may I add. When no one was looking, I just had to tenderly squeeze that plump, black, scaly body. The big lizard didn't seem to mind one bit and some of those so-called experts are always handling the creatures in the name of science, aren't they?

The facts are that visitors to the Galapagos Islands are very seldom compelled to touch the animals through fear of not knowing what the animal's response would be. And very few visitors are dense enough to single out young and pet those same young in front of protective parents.

Back in Puerto Ayora, a very personal natural ecological singularity began to unravel. The room cleaner to my hotel room had snitched on me when seeing some bathroom tissue floating guiltily in the toilet pan. Hence, I was instructed by a slightly bossy receptionist that I had to dispose of used tissue in the little bathroom bin. Doing sign language by pretending to blow my nose, it was then asked via this demonstration, did this mean used tissues too (I will let the imagination run wild as to the other demonstration I could have performed). Needless to say, I am not what one would call pusillanimous (a pussy) so some grace was saved by pointing out that there was no notice on the hotel room wall stating the rules regarding paper disposal.

I don't like to be told off, you know.

The bigger question that needs posing is why human effluent flows into the sea per se? Are you telling me that we cannot devise huge underground vats to dissolve human waste?

Floreana Island was the next stop in my Galapagos voyage (laborious). Just as I began to wonder if this Galapagos lark was worth all the hassle, after being seated uncomfortably in another speeding-like passenger boat, a huge whale's tail was witnessed jutting out of the ocean depth, juxtaposed with a school of blue dolphin who escorted us into the bay.

Human history and being told about eccentric Germans having babies in caves by a tour guide was not what I had travelled 6,163 (as the crow flies) miles for. Unless the baby was still there in the cave, of course. What was learnt at Floreana was that wasps (aggressive ones too) are not really attracted to perfumes or suchlike but attracted to colours we could be wearing, like yellow and orange. Moreover, we were advised that if one of those bad-tempered jaspers rested on our bare arm, to gently blow on it (easier said than done), instead of panicking and running around like a screaming lunatic. It was also advised to not wear garish bright jewellery when snorkelling or diving, which could attract the attention of inquiring sharks.

A few very important lessons were learnt in Floreana; in that you are right to trust your instinct in being sceptical when the experts say in those daft guide books that the Galapagos waters are 'warm in May'. After dipping in my big toe and going on the reports of other bathers, the waters around the Galapagos can have multiple currents, at different temperatures, including very cold. The rocks are also treacherous, and those waves can toss you onto the imposing sharp black stones to disable the strongest of swimmers into limp, bleeding rag dolls.

One older gentleman was literally brought to his knees when testing the power of the Pacific Ocean at Floreana. Having donned himself in all the wet suit regalia, the waves had flipped him onto the rocks so casually, but with such an unpredictable menace, that he crawled out on to the littoral literally on his knees. The tour guide and concerned members of his group then rushed to his aid. He had underestimated the capricious power of the sea and nearly paid with his life.

Last but not least, at Floreana I witnessed my first, dead, washed-up sea-urchin. Although not an outlandish creature to some, I personally find them amazing. Did you know that this UFO (Unidentified Floating Object) can live beyond 200 years?

Pinzon, to the west of Santa Cruz, is another two-hour speed-boat ride (gruelling). Progressive adjectives to describe the travelling aside, to see the blue-footed boobies dive at 60mph like arrows into the ocean (for fish), and for a curious baby seal to swim to the boat was quite remarkable.

I was participating in a reality TV docudrama and seeing it all through my own personal lens.

On the way to Pinzon, and by now being eagle-eyed, I spotted a long piece of submerged floating plastic on which blinked an eye. It was the trumpet species, one would later learn, a very odd fish indeed. Nevertheless, such was the travel rivalry back at the hotel, when I relayed my plastic fish story (some guests try to outdo each other with regard to who has been where and seen what) one young Swedish traveller tried to spoil that special moment between the fish and me by uttering a nonchalant comment as if to indicate seeing a trumpet fish was commonplace. Not for me it wasn't. I later pointed out that everyone staying at our cheapish hostel was a big fish in the travelling stakes (to keep with the fishy plastic story) even those who had visited obscure countries like Paraguay. At the hotel-cum-hostel, stories were relayed to me regarding those who give up everything to travel the world long-term, to then realise a few weeks in that it is not for them and they return home. We all want to feel that sense of calm adventure by exploring the unknown, to help understand what's around us and what will become of us. Travel is to the betterment of all.

Tortuga Bay will no doubt be introduced when staying at Puerto Ayora, which by all accounts is a good trek inland from shore. Let your imagination run wild as you walk along, I say, in picturing the first settlers brandishing those long swords tearing a human path into the harsh landscape. It was at the beach on Tortuga Bay that one of the most intriguing quandaries of the trip presented. I eyed the cackling lava gull drop a crab from mid-air and went over to investigate. Subsequently, I then went into crouch position behind the crab and facing the gull (who showed little fear of me). The gull had already eaten two of the crab's legs and was not about to give up the rest of its meal. What would you do in this situation, toss the still-alive crab back into the sea or let the gull finish its meal because it's just nature? It wouldn't be just nature if we were the poor old crab now, would it? If I were the crab in this random scheme we call life, I would have pleaded with that kind gentleman to save me, opting to desperately hobble around minus two legs for the rest of my days, and so would you.

I left the beach area and did not interfere, deducing that I had already seen the gull peck at the body part of the crab beforehand, which could have fatally wounded it. I was not sure if the crab would in fact survive with two legs missing.

Talking of dead animals, the strip, where tourists gorge on seafood is also worth a mention, especially those giant cockroach-like grey lobsters (langoustines).

Hope you enjoyed your sea insects, people.

The untouchable North Seymour would be my final voyage. This time around, the trip was short, calm and casual (it cost a little more, £150, perhaps that's the reason why) and was a breeze in comparison to the other trips. The guests were even welcomed onboard with a glass of something sparkling.

After perusing images taken of me on North Seymour, one had to muse if David Attenborough could inadvertently turn his hair nest-like when visiting? It's a wonder that the blue-footed boobies and frigates on this island didn't start scrapping for who could nest in Kev's wild, windswept barnet, I say.

Intriguing fossilised skeletal frames of a baby seal and an iguana were also well-spotted on North Seymour. However, when the tour guide was asked how the baby seal had died he said it was because humans had touched it (or something like). What poppycock. As stated previously, nobody with half a brain would have gone near those seals, especially with the non-gregarious ma and pa seal standing guard.

We were then casually informed by the same tour guide that land iguanas have two penises. The frigates (those birds with the big red iridescent balloons under their beak signifying they were advertising for a mate) did not disappoint either.

On the return, two American snorkelling enthusiasts enthused regarding the octopuses they had seen that changed colour to camouflage themselves. They also described (after my prompting) that they had borne witness to eight-inch-long seahorses off Isabela.

How fascinating is that?

To finalise this once in ten lifetimes' Ecuadorian experience, it would be a human, not an animal drama which would feature as an endnote. Nonchalantly boarding the ferry to reach Baltra for the flight home, having casually forgotten to retrieve my suitcase from the bus, blind panic set in. Remembering that I had exchanged a few sentences with a young and very pleasant Mexican lady on that initial bus ride, who spoke very good English, I quickly and efficiently explained my plight to her as we alighted the ferry, just as another bus awaited to take us on to the final leg of the airport sequence home.

She was immediately on the case, which saw me returning to the mainland on a ferry of my own. As I neared, I could see the bus still parked, but had visions of it pulling out at any time, complete with my case.

Frantically searching the bus to see that the case had gone, others had noticed the kerfuffle and one local directed me to my luggage which was sitting outside one of those portable kiosks.

The moral to this endnote is that it's always wise to factor in that extra bit of time for your flight in case of unforeseen circumstances. If I had not factored in that extra time, I would have had to choose between missing my flight to Guayaquil, Amsterdam and Manchester, which would have set me back a few thousand pounds, or to forego my luggage (if I had my passport on my person, of course).

I never did like that light turquoise, easily stainable, travel case you know.

Let them Eat Cake

Finally, it appears, we can have an honest debate regarding our unexceptional royal family without being accused of treason and holed up in the Tower. I will admit, point blank, that I believe the monarchy should be abolished and we should elect a head of state and change the national anthem to be more class/culturally inclusive.

Will I lose my head for making such a bold statement?

I would never sing the national anthem. *God save our gracious queen*? How absurd. If there was a God why would he/she want to save somebody who lives an opulent selfish lifestyle while their subjects face abject poverty and resort to foodbanks?

Sorry, don't buy it.

Then we have the hangers-on like Prince Andrew and that brassy flame-haired toe-sucker, Fergie. Associating with billionaire paedophiles and cavorting with broods of corrupt North African despots have been the essence of another royal PR disaster for those two liabilities.

It's also worth pointing out that in the years leading up to the Second World War, our Lizzie and Co had close associations with the Nazi regime.

And whoever said the monarchy was separate from the state was a born liar. Not only do our soldiers swear an allegiance to the queen before they go into battle, the so-called politically themed Palace of Westminster is no more than a seat of banal royal regalia.

Personally, I found the tour of the Palace of Westminster largely nauseating. Royalist propaganda dictated amidst tacky splendour was forced in my face from start to finish. I had purposely chosen Westminster because of political interest and would have opted for Buckingham Palace if that way inclined.

More to the point, how can the monarchy maintain neutrality from the state when Charles becomes king? He has meddled in just about every political event over the years via his 'obedient servants' (as signed off by one Labour MP).

Has anybody else noticed how some people sort of sigh with respect and smile reverently when conversing regarding the royal family? They argue that the monarchy is not parasitic; but brings in the bacon for the country and London would not have as many tourists without them. In fact, Queen Elizabeth II is the legal owner of about 6,600 million acres of land and the only person on earth who owns whole countries. The value of her land holding is approximately **£17,600,000,000,000**. A lot of zeros, isn't it?

That being said, Princess Diana did do some good work regarding Aids sufferers in the 1980s, but so could an elected head of state who didn't spend £2,000 a week on makeup. It is not treasonable or discourteous to describe myself as an English republican who believes our four home countries should become independent, minus the monarchy.

Our royal family has also an unsavoury and questionable history, hasn't it? We had the warring three sons of Queen Victoria, instrumental in starting the First World War, where millions perished. In fact, in 1917 the royals changed their family name to Windsor from the German Saxe-Coburg and Gotha, due to anti-German sentiment brought about by the war.

Talking of surnames, our monarchy's original surname was the incongruous Battenberg but was then changed to the more Anglicised Mountbatten, again because of anti-German sentiment during the period.

Brings a whole new meaning to the phrase 'Let them eat cake', doesn't it?

Change Comes in Threes

Times are a-changing and the rubric regarding those being elected has shifted in dramatic mode. We can first start with Labour leader Jeremy Corbyn and the demeaning bile wasted on him by the print press in the run-up to the May 2017 general election. Yours truly was one of the few who declared in writing (Twitter) that unelected Prime Minister Theresa May was not liked (her sour, quaquaversal facial expressions don't help) and if she dropped any more clangers, like the social care gaffe, and factoring in Corbyn's popular scrapping tuition fees policy, it could be a hung parliament. It appears that it is of no significance what the controlling asinine media want anymore, social media has put paid to that. The state comptrollers have lost their influence. Regarding the eventual deal made with the DUP for the Tories to stay in government, even hardened loyal Conservatives are uncomfortable with it. Only time will tell on that one, time May hasn't got.

Then of course there was the political earthquake stateside in November 2016 with the election of Donald Trump. Does anybody seriously believe those Russian fairy tale chapters concocted by the 'Fake News'? Trump has ticked some plus boxes in bringing the fake news concept into focus; the news corporations have been faking it here since transmission. Taking the controlling news corporations on, and not losing, has been a great undertaking for Trump, never mind the building of the wall. We do understand that drug dealing gangsterism has almost had a free rein, but to build the Great Wall of Texas as a restrictive? Whatever one may think of Trump, just look at the alternative – Hillary Clinton. Clinton and her emails aside, health care, gun laws and 'Jerusalem' (and no, I'm not an anti-Semite) could prove costly for Trump; a two-state solution in bringing Palestine in from the cold for round table talks and affordable health care for all has to be the way forward for civilised societies.

Then we had Trump's childish bickerings with North Korea. We have an expression in these parts, Mr Trump, it goes: "Don't talk about it do it." Trump, however, did just that on June 12th 2018 (Singapore) by meeting with Kim Jong-un, leader of North Korea. The first meeting between US and North Korean leaders was a massive success, but pilloried by the liberal elite, who bellyached that there was no detail to the agreement. A warmongering climate suits some, you know.

I am not arguing that our national media is over reporting the by now, 'old news' as detailed above. But all the BBC/Sky News affiliations (they report on exactly the same stories at exactly the same time) seem to have wanted to report on through the years 2017 and 2018 is: Trump, Brexit, Trump, Brexit, Trump, Brexit or Brexit–Trump, Brexit, Brexit, Brexit. All this, when as a nation, we are regressing politically, socially and culturally. Imagine the delight on Newsnight then, when the BBC managed to secure their two favourite topics – Brexit and Trump at one fell scoop, in that Trump hinted there would be no trade deal with the US if there was to be a soft Brexit. Yes, those paid propagandists not only frothed at the bit, but alarmingly failed to air the other side to the argument. Is this because representatives from the Republican Party and/or the Brexit camp will not volunteer for an interview with the mainstream media, such is their naked bias. Or is social media now the mainstream, which is the reason why there are calls from the media giants to curtail it, arguing it contains fake news? Challenging times or what. Then we had that historically recherché summit between Trump and Putin held in Helsinki on July 16th 2018. You would not have thought so though by the hysterical reaction from the world media. A rare chance for world peace, the liberal elite groaned like never seen before, but this time in baleful tones. The BBC, CH 4, Sky, Fox, CNN, you name it were all visibly upset, hurt, betrayed, angry and even distraught. Yes, the bitterness was tangible. The battle for the US appears to be between government and the intelligence services (who have always controlled the West). It can be disseminated that neither will claim a victory. Why?

Because it will be ordinary voters who will eventually triumph. The tide has already turned. It has to be said that more and more 'ordinaries' are beginning to respect Donald Trump. Even those who sit firmly on the 'social conscience' side of politics. Who else would blatantly rip up those diplomatic World Order conventions we are all so disgusted by – giving them both barrels in the process?

Take NATO (North Atlantic Treaty Organisation) for example, many in Britain agree with Trump that NATO is an ineffective and expensive waste of time.

Conversely, the Republican Party (as well as most political commentators world-wide) appear to be obsessed with the mythical 'left'. Some would argue that there was, and is, no such thing. To dig a little deeper regarding the 'left' myth, how else should we refer to those principled with human grace and fairness? Are critics who use the word 'left' not referring to the socially moral, but tacitly denoting those over liberal or ultra-politically correct? In early November 2018, days before the US Midterm elections, we saw televised tit-for-tat exchanges between Obama and Trump; with Trump talking about far-left judges featuring in the Obama years. Far-left judges? You're having a laugh – nothing effectively changed for the majority of US citizens during the Obama administration, far-left judges or not, so what was the far-left point about, immigration? Clarification is needed; politics is mixed-up enough.

As with the 'left' misconception, the same goes for the 'right'. I would therefore assert that there is no such thing as right and left in politics anymore. Voters, today, hand-pick policy from all parties and then come to a decision on who to cast their vote for accordingly.

They say it comes in threes. Well the decision by the British people to vote for Brexit was a mammoth event. Some of us did predict the result because we understand how ordinary English people feel in being left out of mainstream politics. Apparently, 53.4 % of the voters in England voted for Brexit, while 46.6 % voted against. In the north however, the figure rose to 68% for and 32% against. This is a crystal clear and decisive majority. It was not enough for many MPs and other establishment figures though, apparently for some, the British people did not know what they were doing, or they were not informed of the full implications/facts, so there should be another referendum. Others, like the Lib Dems, jumped on pro-EU sentiment because they have nothing else to offer the electorate after being in bed with Tories for five years, complicit in forcing austere misery on the population

It could be true to say that sections of both Leave and Remain supporters believe that the EU (European Union) is an elitist, establishmentarian and corrupt institution and ordinary people are no better off because of it. The argument to fight for EU reform by remaining inside bears no weight – it has not changed in over forty years, so it's not going to change now. The overly bureaucratic EU will only consider reforming when member states begin to pull out.

Britain voted to pull out.

Chairing the Member and the Political Sixth Sense

The Sir John Soane's Museum in London is well worth a visit, especially when Hogarth's *Chairing the Member* portrait is uncovered. This portrait highlights some very interesting metaphors indeed. One of the four Humours of an Election series completed in 1755, *Chairing the Member* echoes the same interpretation as can be seen today.

First of all, it is common knowledge that the generic *Chairing the Member* image is depicting corruption pervasive amongst the privileged classes in Oxfordshire in the 18th century, namely the Whigs and the Tories (one of the same) who were the only political parties in operation between the 1680s and the 1850s. Ring any bells for today? I'll give you a clue: the Labour/Conservative parties and the misuse of expenses.

Now let's single out the characters in the picture and work out their significance. Turning back in time, without over-Labouring the point, we have a blind fiddler leading the junket. Rhyming alongside, the focal point pageant also captures a successful Tory candidate about to be toppled. I would go one further by saying that the goose flying overhead (perhaps off to warmer climes) is about to drop one (a golden egg that is) to land on that unsuspecting privileged bonce as a sort of retribution for wanton corpulence, which brings a whole new twist to the fable *Killing the Goose that laid the Golden Egg*.

Moreover, in Hogarth's masterpiece we can bear witness to a group of frightened pigs running across the scene, apparently in reference to the story of the 'Gadarene Swine'. To me this one's obvious; if it were an up-to-date referent, the hogs would be symbolising those from England who trooped north across the border to grunt 'No' to Scotland's independence referendum of 2014. Insomuch as none were more repellent than George Galloway attempting to save his own bacon, having been elected by the UK and unionist dynamic. Didn't you know, George, that the premise which underpins socialist values (you being a socialist and all) is non-imperialistic? The 1707 Act of Union which enabled England to dominate Scotland (which saw the enabling of the 'UK') was imperialism at its worst; so why do you think Galloway was so eager for unionism to prevail instead of supporting Scottish self-determination?

Back to Hogarth's masterpiece, the ordinary classes amassed at the front of the chapel as the backdrop suggests that the electorate don't know how to mobilise politically, but are attempting to organise in a fashion. To the left of the painting we can see servitude epitomised by servile serfs supplying luxury goods to those of a covetous disposition to gorge on. We would probably call them jobsworths today.

There can also be seen amidst the pandemonium a subtle allegory of the five senses: Fiddler (hearing), Fainting Woman (smell), Bear (taste), Chair Bearer (touch) and Spectacles (sight).

Albeit, the real meaning behind Hogarth's *Chairing the Member* could be the sixth sense (political awareness) parable. In that by his painting, Hogarth was prophesying that by acquiring a political sixth sense the masses would eventually fine tune and coordinate their constitutional reach to topple the opulent ruling elite once and for all.

Imagine Liverpool's John Lennon Airport Accessible

I thought I had secured a bargain in September 2017; the bargain being a £72 return trip from Liverpool to Madrid. Atletico and Real here we come.

But all did not meet the eye – so to Speke.

Things just seemed a little back to front when purchasing my rail ticket because I discovered that I would have to travel south from Stoke to Stafford to head north to Liverpool.

My taxi came at 12.15pm to take me to Stoke-on-Trent railway station. The journey from Stoke to Stafford took twenty minutes and I then had to wait at Stafford for fifteen minutes for the train north to Liverpool South Parkway (one hour). Then it was the turn of the shuttle bus which took another twenty minutes from South Parkway to the airport to travel back south again on to Madrid. Unbelievable isn't it?

Things were about to get worse.

I have never been so alarmed at the poor operations policy coupled with disastrous customer services offered by the well-known 'budget' airline I was travelling with.

When I first arrived at the airport in good time, the departures board stated that the flight would be departing at 18.25 instead of 17.10. When you see a delay on the departures board you have that gut feeling that the delay could escalate, and this particular airline did not disappoint. After going through to board at around 18.30, we were ushered through one section where we had to produce our passports. Then we just stood there after filing through the gate because of an 'operational' difficulty. Apparently, they were waiting for more staff.

At this point those that have trouble standing for a long time would have to suffer as a result. One passenger registered disabled with chronic pain syndrome found it distressing standing for so long. This person did not like to make their disability known and compromise another passenger, in that the passenger would have to give up their sitting space, so they suffered in silence. Airline staff should not have let us through in the first place, this was an unprofessional and, some would say, negligent decision. In effect, we were forced to stand and did not have the option to sit if we wanted to.

It was then announced that they were again 'waiting for staff to arrive' which sounded disingenuous, considering they had previously stated that it was an operational or technical problem. We must have stood there for between forty-five minutes and one hour, to be taken on board the aircraft, where the pilot said we would have to wait another thirty minutes for another member of staff to turn up. He said the reason for the initial delay was previous high winds in relation to a flight from Amsterdam, which had affected this flight. This knock-on effect had nothing to do with our flight, I would later argue. Under regulation (EC) No. 261/2004, airlines are liable for a delay of three hours or more but can maintain that the delay was out of their control if it was due to inclement weather. The weather was perfectly temperate in Liverpool and Madrid so they weren't going to play that one, I reasoned. We then waited another forty-five minutes to one hour on the aircraft for a member of staff to arrive. Pre-arrival, all the cabin crew had offered as a sweetener was to dish up cheap plastic cups of water instead of issuing us with refreshment vouchers as stipulated in the airline's policy.

At Madrid airport, I then had to get a taxi, which cost thirty euros, when I had planned to get the metro. With being delayed for so long and disorientated as a result, I even forgot to ask the taxi driver for a receipt.

Let's recap: I had initially set off from Newcastle-under-Lyme at 12.15pm for the flight to Madrid and subsequently arrived at my hotel in Madrid at around 1am, which was some thirteen hours later. This is not acceptable; you can get to the moon and back quicker.

It was all smiles on the return flight from Madrid to Liverpool, I observed. There was almost a spring in the step of the airline staff as if they had been briefed to mete out special customer treatment for the disgruntled, there were probably claims on the way too. The Scousers know their rights, you know.

I was amused that we even set off for the runway before the designated flight departure time, which must have been a first.

We sort of efficiently glided back to Merseyside, arriving bang on time.

The nightmare was not yet over though.

I had not anticipated the length of the walk from the aircraft to customs and never expected such queues to get through those customs. I then had to wait half an hour in the cold outside Liverpool Airport for a bus to shuttle me to Liverpool South Parkway again, to wait on a cold waiting room-less platform for another thirty minutes for the train to Stafford, to then wait twenty minutes at Stafford railway station to arrive at Stoke at 11.25pm.

We are in the travel dark ages, I am afraid to inform you.

Therefore, is the airline in question putting customers off from flying from Liverpool Airport, when factoring in the distance from Liverpool South Parkway to the airport and the repeated changes/waiting for connections endured for access? Should the airlines using the airport not be liaising with Liverpool City Council to finance rapid transport access directly onto the concourse?

Then to top it all, I had the punishing delay seeing me quiescent for some three hours fifteen minutes, not because of aircraft/airport technicalities, but through staffing problems. Personally, I feel as though I would not opt to travel from Liverpool Airport again.

To zoom in on the carriers underscored, there are other far-reaching conclusions to be drawn from the delay shenanigans. The truth is that I did not feel safe travelling with this particular airline if they can offer such a shambolic unprofessional customer service experience such as the one outlined.

Liverpool John Lennon Airport? Imagine all the people travelling from A to B efficiently.

It isn't hard to do. No need to travel north to head south. And face unprecedented delays too.

Note: In October 2018 I flew to Madrid again, this time from Birmingham International Airport. Although there was a one-hour delay outbound, and I had to endure that appalling 'packed like a sardine' Cross Country rail experience, I did manage to secure the most unusual photograph; taken during my first ever flamenco show (see centre pages).

Good Riddance to Bad Rubbish

The shocking announcement in the summer of 2011 by James Murdoch (son of Rupert) that the *News of the World* (*NOTW*) was to discontinue with immediate effect was met with suspicion by many. The last edition would also be advertisement empty and its profits would be donated to charity.

By all accounts, the spotlight had now been cleverly taken off the paper since it does not exist; not to mention all the bribery and corruption associated with the brand. The *Sun* newspaper then followed up, and highlighted stories gained from the same *NOTW* journalists who hacked the phones of Milly Dowler, the Soham girls, and our dead soldiers' families, and as so, is just as blameworthy.

There were also rumours circulating that the *NOTW* would be sold under a new guise, such as the *Sunday Sun*, which brought on a whole new sense of disgust to those actively criticising media ethics. As staff at the *NOTW* trooped out of the Wapping plant to a round of applause anybody would have thought they had been engaged over the years in something admirable. Many were expecting them to hang their heads in shame.

As the media mogul himself, Rupert Murdoch, arrived at News International sporting a straw boater and apparently reading the last copy of the *NOTW*, already the focus seemed to have shifted regarding the culture of newspapers like this. In its final edition we were drowned by crass sentimentality in the form of 'the better readers' comments, coupled by a strange cherry-picked montage of former front pages highlighting pioneering stories like the exposé of dishonesty within the Pakistani cricket team.

What about all the cheap, made up, sensationalist and downright sick stories propagated by this tacky tabloid relating to murder victims and their families? What about the disgusting lies told regarding Hillsborough and the sexualising of children as seen with the disappearance of Madeleine McCann? What about the glorification of murderers (where this newspaper has generated interest in these monsters as some kind of titillating read) and what about *NOTW* journalists deleting the messages on Milly Dowler's phone so the family were duped into believing she could still be alive?

The *NOTW* always purported to be a family newspaper but successively published sordid sex scandal after sordid sex scandal; then there were the veiled threats that if politicians spoke out against the paper the *NOTW* would 'come after them' and publish details of their personal lives. Yes, they were nasty bullies too and ruthlessly profiteered from it all.

Then we had the subtle conditioning of readers that celebrity culture is the be-all and end-all of existence. Readers were saturated with it. And what about influencing people on how to think and vote?

Just when we thought the depravity depths of the phone hacking scandal could not sink any lower, it was revealed that together with victims of the 7/7 bombings, during their darkest hours, the families of our dead military personnel may have had their phones hacked too. All this in order to publish salacious follow-up stories to sensationalise the victim's tragedy and rubbish the family's grief.

What is also alarming is that the chief executive of News International, Rebekah Brooks, had not stepped down on the orders of media mogul Rupert Murdoch. It got worse: Prime Minister David Cameron had been seen to be entertaining 'in it up to his neck' former *NOTW* editor Andrew Coulson at 10 Downing Street. After shock revelation after shock revelation, we did see most of our MPs discover their backbone for the first time in their political lives as they formed orderly queues to attack the Murdoch empire monopoly in an emergency debate, but the outraged general public wants more.

They don't want celebrities and politicians with a private axe to grind against journalists to clean up in claims regarding these revelations. They have enough money. It could be true to say that any monies received from the tabloids to the celebrities in compensation should be used to set up a new Press Standards Commission with full powers. At present, the Press Complaints Commission is impotent because it is run by the media barons themselves (how can we have themselves investigating themselves?). The public also wanted to see the Metropolitan Police (who had been releasing crime information for cash payment) and the press, investigated by an outside body with a view to the high profile players receiving long prison sentences.

Judging by the smirking faces of both Murdoch and Brooks leaving a swanky Mayfair restaurant around this time, they obviously knew something which we didn't that gave rise to such relaxed body language (maybe it's the fact that it was going to be business as usual because those on high had already exonerated them of any wrongdoing).

Like Labour leader Ed Miliband had previously exclaimed regarding Cameron and Co, 'they just don't get it' do they? They just don't get how incensed ordinary people are regarding the whole culture of the media industry, especially the print press. Perhaps the fear of a stint on remand at Brixton and Holloway, for Murdoch and Brooks respectively, would have wiped the stupid grins from their faces. But they got off the hook and Coulson assumed the fall guy role.

If Murdoch and Brooks were not complicit in widespread duplicity at the *NOTW*, or they knew nothing about it; then they are not in touch with the mechanics of their businesses and so Murdoch is not fit to run BSkyB or any other media conglomerate.

My Journey to the Centre of the Earth

In introduction, I must apologise for using the word journey. I loathe the word. This is because those who aspire to the privileged class are always 'on journeys' (or jarneees) of some sort, aren't they?

My only experience of the mining industry is as a child, living in the former Forest Park area of Hanley, which displayed the 'Devil's chimneys'. The chimneys were black fissures in the hot earth encasing red burning embers. It was caused by Hanley Deep Pit.

During my childhood I was aware of the natural secure warm glow which could only be associated with the coal fire, having fetched a shovel of coal or even slack from the coal bunker or the coal house on many occasions.

I was always a dab hand with the poker, too, and knew how to make and then 'draw' a coal fire by placing a sheet of newspaper around the fireguard.

Similarly, I have never been reticent to relay that both my father and grandfathers were miners. In saying that, nebulous second-hand titbits regarding local pit disasters, dust diseases, blackouts and strikes of the 1970s and 1980s respectively, about sums up my mining knowledge.

A visit to the Apedale Heritage Centre in Chesterton was about to change all that.

It has to be said that I speak as I find and am not easily impressed or influenced, being both cynical and critical if the situation demands.

Although the museum is free to peruse, the tour of the Apedale Colliery cost £6 in 2015 (with informative guides) and lasted between forty-five minutes to an hour.

And yes, I did feel a bit of a nit wearing the hard hat, but let me tell you I was glad of it later on in the tour, considering I bumped my head twice underground.

Historically speaking and right up to this day, although it was backbreaking work mining the innermost recesses of the earth (where some of the men even toiled naked, such was the heat) there is much more to the colliers' story.

Mineworkers would need to equip themselves with the appropriate geoscience. As well as coal seams and other rock formations to learn about, there are theories around funnelling the air supply together with managing gases like methane (firedamp) carbon dioxide (blackdamp) and the odourless carbon monoxide. There is also the prerequisite of needing to understand timers and explosives (like dynamite) to dislodge the obstinate black rock. Then there are the miles of underground tunnels that would have to be navigated, where conveyers, children and even horses have assisted in excavating the tonnage.

For my part, the most telling snippet of data acquired during the visit was that coal is the product of millions of years-old decomposed tree, plant and swamp matter. Who would have thought that?

Today there is serious discourse surrounding the reopening of some specialist mines for clean fuel burning. It should also be considered that we still import coal of different variations from abroad.

If the reopening policy should bring about sustainable employment for future generations, I am all for it. The underground education, as described above, concurs with a worthwhile and sought-after profession for those drawn to the industry.

To the contrary, there is a concern that if we were to keep mining the earth in ever larger quantities (thus interfering with the natural geological infrastructure) it will ultimately cause an imbalance. This could result in tremors as experienced over the years, especially in the North Staffordshire area.

Therefore, could those mini-quakes ever escalate into something of a greater magnitude?

To conclude the tour, 'a splendid education' best illustrates the encounter, even though I only scratched the coal surface, so to speak.

More importantly, to be mindful of the myth regarding the miner being propagated as an uneducated blackened-faced labourer will help avoid fool's gold-like mistakes with job description identity in later life.

Which is probably the most important lesson to be learnt of all.

Niagara Falls

It is not comical to say that those living in social housing have to endure toilet noises comparable to Niagara Falls due to ruthless speculators cutting costs on soundproofing. You see, to live in peace and quiet in a soundproofed home is a fundamental human right, so why do you think housing associations do not allow for this right? Better soundproofed homes would be less of a strain on the police force too, who are called out to countless domestics, sparked off by loud appliances that could be muted with decent acoustics.

Question: what's the definition of a slum? Answer: Everyone knows deep down if they are living in a contemporary slum.

There are countless residents in social housing today that know all about the modern slum.

Then there are the fire issues; heavy fire doors can stop the smoke getting to the fire alarm in the hall, so if there was a fire, you would be dead before the smoke alarm sounded. But if you dared to pose this and other concerns to the fire service, some fire service representatives can baffle you with fire science and report every conversation to the social landlord – it's called institutional collusion.

Additionally, the modern British social landlord's favourite tenant frustration is to call damp and mould condensation.

It's all about money, isn't it?

Let's analyse the profits made by the social landlord, where it goes, and what the board members help themselves to with emoluments. Yes, it's nice pickings, if you are allowed to pick, of course. Those living under the cheap umbrella operating by the name of the 'social landlord' expect nothing and are constantly frustrated at being met with housing officers trained in giving nothing.

What is wrong with these jumped-up officials, you might ask? This is people's lives we are talking about.

Then of course housing associations can pass the buck in other ways; their scrooge-like housing laws can come under the remit of the local council, which allows the building contractors to cut back on soundproofing to reduce cost and maximise profit. Sometimes housing complexes are part-financed by local councils. They're in it together.

The latest golden egg or nice little earner for the social landlord is shared accommodation for the elderly. Will any prospective new tenants only be accepted if they are hard of hearing? Then they won't have to suffer the indignity of hearing their neighbours urinate, Niagara Falls style.

"Not Saxon but Celtic"
say Experts

The Saxon Hoard excavated in South East Staffordshire in 2009 could in fact be Celtic, say archaeologists from the internationally-renowned Institute of Trooth. Expert Weeno Moore from the Institute said yesterday:

"The spiral decoration on the pectoral cross is very similar to that seen in treasure found from the Bronze age hundreds of years earlier. The latest carbon dating suggests that the treasure could in fact be Celtic and not Saxon. There is no conclusive evidence that the treasure unearthed near Lichfield did not belong to the Cornovii tribe. In other words: we just don't know."

The revelation has had dignitaries in Stoke-on-Trent reeling, many of whom had earmarked funds for the construction of an 80-foot Saxon warrior to celebrate the find. One local said on hearing the news:

"Erecting that monstrous giant Saxon effigy in North Staffordshire to signify Saxon treasure found in South Staffordshire and it's not even Saxon treasure? It defies belief, even by our standards. I have often been disappointed by the lack of Celtic history at the Potteries Museum. It's as if historians don't want to recognise that the Olde English ever existed as a cultural and economic force. That Saxon find was exhumed in South Staffs, where they talk with a Birmingham accent. More Celtic Staffordshire please."

Update from the Celtic Soothsayer (September 2017).

"Local, your wish for more Celtic Staffordshire has been granted. In Leek, North Staffordshire in December 2016, beautiful Celtic jewellery, which is some 2,500 years old and of an international calibre, was discovered by two metal detecting enthusiasts. Julia Farley of the British Museum has declared

that the find features some of the oldest examples of Celtic ornament ever found in Britain. What will give you the most satisfaction though, local, is the fact that although the Staffordshire Hoard was worth a few bob, the Leekfrith Iron Age torcs are older and worth far more because they were found in your local area, not near to Birmingham. Perhaps your local dignitaries should now consider erecting a giant Celtic warrior queen beside the A500 in Stoke. For impact, she could be clutching a severed head."

As an addendum to the warrior queen idea: On the 19th November 2018, Caistor St Edmund (Venta Iscenoru) in Norfolk was visited – the very same spot which oversaw the Iceni revolt against Roman rule in AD60. Although it was not feasible to capture a glimpse of Boudica in person, I did manage a stunning image to befit the scene (see centre pages).

Food for Thought

With poverty deepening for many, it is food for thought that, while the bankers still take millions, energy companies continually hike prices and politicians mock by preaching penny-pinching virtues, as a people we are unable to challenge the system we are controlled by.

To best understand this enigma, perhaps we have to look back to the late 18th century, when English children were deposed from the horrors of the parish workhouses in the south, to the heinous cotton mills of the north, to face unimaginable horrors.

In that era, in a society governed by the hierarchy, even the lowest paupers ascribed to a pecking order.

Those with families looked down on the orphans, elders looked down on the younger and bastards were reviled by all. Simultaneously, the lower classes looked up to and would have gladly taken the place of their privileged enslavers. When the children were sold to the mills they were lured by their own aspirations to subjugate others like they had been subjugated themselves.

The parish authorities that presided over the workhouses promised the children nobility, standing, money, and roast beef and plum pudding every day when they were relocated and took their rightful place as a noble. Naturally it was a ruse, but on hearing the news and believing their salvation had come, the impoverished children assumed the character of the upper classes as they swaggered about, lauding it up, now refusing to bow down to the overseers of the workhouse.

This tragic enactment begs an interesting question; is the real reason the class system has survived for centuries because we aspire to be what our masters are? Or is the premise of suffering from the affliction of having no backbone inherently an English disease? This can be best answered by a situation that arose in Rouen in 1812. When one of the English cotton mill tyrants tried to impose the inhumane cotton mill regulations onto the French factory workers, a strike was called and the army called in.

In saying that, in more recent times, even the French have been battened down with backward and retrogressive working conditions.

Where does that leave us?

A Letter to Cameron (2015)

Dear Dave

I have spoken to you in a couple of my previous articles and was most disappointed you did not respond; especially when you were live on *Question Time*. I can read code inferences, you know (especially the Freemasons, wink wink).

Talking of *Question Time*, it was a jolly good show, Dave. However, I must confess that you need some advice from yours truly if you want to become elected again (by a majority, of course). In that eventuality I want to formerly make a request to become your personal stylist and confidant (I've been around the block a few times, Dave, and can brief you on how to keep those pesky peasants conditioned).

Don't think I didn't notice that trendy flick-like quiff on the front of your wig (perhaps Stacey the stylist is finally listening to my advice). That mod style suits you, Dave, and will appeal not just to the voting pensioners, but to the under-fifties as well. On the other hand (or should I say head), I could have sworn I saw a little thatched patch as that nasty cameraman swivelled around to the rear to expose that delicate hair deficiency you are managing. Have you been eating your crusts, Dave?

Hey, that was a good one when you pulled that crumpled piece of paper out of your jacket pocket; what did it say again regarding the bankrupt treasury you inherited? "There's no money left." Are you sure it was not a letter from the MPs' expenses office, Dave? After all, duck ponds don't come cheap, you know.

I have to say it's been Billy Blunder after Billy Blunder during the campaign because I haven't been there to advise you. The West Ham clanger took the biscuit. Anyway, I know and you know, you know your working man's sports, Dave. And how many times have I told you to affix that mask on tight so it doesn't slip?

You did have the female voters swooning though, Dave, when you rolled up your sleeves on that freshly laundered shirt (hope you used Ariel, Dave and not that working class Daz). What a lather you got in, frenziedly foaming to propagate your economic policies again. Don't take your shirt off though, Dave, like the grafters do, and if Ned challenges you to bare-chested fisticuffs, like the old days at Eton, have some decorum and walk away. No decent blue-blooded descendant of William IV would lower themselves, Dave. If that state school commoner Mr Ed takes his top off and starts addling with you ignore him because it's all balderdash. He's after more female admirers-come-voters when we all know you are the political heartthrob of this election.

Yes, talking about your economic policies is it two million jobs you, Witchy Poo Treece, IDS (can't say what that stands for Dave in a family manuscript) and Kathy Hepburn sound-alike Willie have created between you? What's more, take no notice of those snipers when they say you are looking after your rich shop-owning chums in the supermarket economy, they're lower than a snake's belly. A few poundlands an hour is perfectly adequate for the serfs, isn't it, Dave? They should be thankful they have got a job. Those scrawmers on the dole need a good hard day's work around their back too. Have 'em working for their bread, Dave, £70 per week dole money is a lot of lolly in Paupersville and enough for anyone to live on – I bet prudent Dave could do it with coppers left over.

Ooh, and when you swore on telly. There's no need for that you know, Dave. I know that potty Boris probably argues that bloody's in the bible, bloody's in the book, if you don't bloody believe me go and bloody look. Watch that Batty Boris, Dave; he's a kibitzer and not as barmy as he makes out, especially where top jobs with top pay packets are at stake.

Another thing, Dave, I know you said you want to see everyone holding that stobby (stubby) pencil in the polling booth for the possible referendum on in/out of Europe, but I was wondering whether the voters will know what they are voting for this time around. You see, that other referendum you cobbled together with that great pretender Sticky Nicky was a little bit of a big fat fib too (keep away from him, Dave, he will have you wearing that same T-shirt again). I don't know about round your way, Dave, but round here, most don't know what proportional representation is, never mind vote for it. As far as we are concerned AV stands for Aston Villa and not West Ham.

Look; yes Dave, all the top politicians are quoting the look word when being put on the spot. Try to say look with an ooh instead, so you don't sound like a repetitive copycat (even that Nigel Pigel Farage is doing it). I know down south you say 'buck' for 'boohk' but polish up your vowels and take some elocution lessons, Dave, and you will appeal to voters both in Birmingham and further north. One, two, three… looohk.

Talking of which, you might scoff at us up north cuz we've got nowt, Dave, and I know you think we still call London 'the Smoke' but how many jobs do yer want? Your little Freudian slip of referring to the May 7th vote as a 'career-defining election' suggests you have further plans for that little boys' club of yours (for he's a jolly good fellow, for he's…).

Dave, there's only two days to go so I will close now to add the finishing touches to your fetching new makeover (win or lose the election). It's called the Malcolm Ally look. Seventies is the new twenty-fifteens according to the fashion gurus you know, Dave. The Marks and Sparks garb you currently sport is so last summer. I was thinking that a black boater, like Ally's, will discreetly cover that little thatch you have got going on (if it gets any worse Dave you could always opt for a Bobby Charlton). Besides, that fur-collared number did not do the former Manchester City boss any harm (psst… you will appear both football savvy and a true blood sports toff) – classless.

Pip pip, Dave.

Little Pidge

The birdbrained thinking of councils across the country that pigeons should be culled to clean up our city centres does not go down well with those who believe the majority of living creatures have a right to exist.

Why are so many disgusted and unnerved by pigeons?

Have we been so conditioned that these little creatures are vermin and 'rats with wings' that we lose all sense of perspective and understanding that pigeons are just foraging in town centres for a bite to eat. They mooch when they have empty stomachs, just like we would do. If it were a parrot or a canary one would not want them culled. Pigeons get a bad press because they are not as aesthetically pleasing as other birds. Is this why some people resent them so much?

From a personal perspective, I can't resent them, even though on one occasion, when eating a baked potato with chilli outside, a pigeon flapped its wings and then flew around me. To my disgust, I then noticed a tiny little mite (insect) in my chilli, obviously shaken from the pigeon's feathers. And no, I did not pick the mite out and carry on eating the jacket.

Children seem to like pigeons unless coerced by their parents or local councils into believing that pigeons are ugly, something to be afraid of, or even dirty. Yes, the pigeon poop can be a tad unsightly, so can dog poo. Talking of dirty council spin, our backward public toilet systems force us to handle taps that have been handled by the not so clean. Not forgetting our antediluvian toilet wiping system when a bidet or water cleaning is far more sanitary-friendly.

What is the council doing about that?

A spokesman from one council has said:

"Pigeons carry Weil's disease, which can cause cardiovascular problems."

Could the council provide further evidence of this, backed up by statistics? In their wisdom, some people in authority (and some members of the general public) would prefer to see the pigeons shot to death in a mass extermination that will not solve the problem entirely. The pigeons will eventually regroup and come back. The derelict buildings all over the country offer a tempting habitat for pigeons to roost and to breed in. Perhaps councils should look at solving the derelict building problem foremost, if they want to make any worthwhile incursion into the pigeon poser.

Where do the council get their moral dispensation to demonise and then to order the butchering of these birds? Why not try to reduce their numbers by making a large section of them infertile? After all, it is done with cats and dogs and even with cockroaches and suchlike, isn't it? Anything has to be better than this blinkered wanton slaughter.

Carrier and homing pigeons saved many human lives during the great world wars, don't forget. Moreover, in other countries (like Nepal) it is believed pigeons bring good luck. The bitter, rat with wings brigade, please note: now you know why you never win anything on the lottery.

Funeral Costs: Prepay and Don't Delay

It's commonplace nowadays for staff at care homes to ask the next of kin the name of the resident's funeral director. For those working in the care system, dealing with death should be included in their job description.

This puts the onus on the living relatives, in that have they made provision for that sad but inevitable consequence?

If they have the capacity, many people nowadays have decided to pre-pay their funeral costs with a funeral bond before the actual event. Furthermore, there are so many pluses for doing so that if you have the finances it would be almost unthinkable not to.

It is not necessarily morbid or depressing to undertake such a task; for some it can be interesting and for others it can even be fun. The biggest incentive must be that the pre-paid price you pay for your funeral is protected against inflation. So if you were to depart this world ten, twenty or even thirty years after planning your own funeral, the cost would remain the same as it was at the time you signed the contract.

Not everyone is insured, though, and many cannot afford funeral costs. Some would even go so far as to say that half-decent funerals are now a preserve of the wealthy.

If you do find yourself in the situation where a loved one has died, and don't have the resources to pay for the funeral, the deceased's relatives must apply to the DWP for the basic costs of a funeral cremation (which is cheaper and known as a pauper's funeral). In this eventuality, living relatives can plead to the DWP for a burial on religious grounds but this will inevitably delay interment. DWP aside, there are many variations in funeral concepts and prices to match. The average cost of a standard funeral without any extras is around the £4,000 figure (2017). There are also cheaper-priced eco-funerals (costing approximately £2,000-£3,000). In addition, the classic horse-drawn carriage can cost up to £1,000, as an extra to the funeral cars, not as a replacement.

Also note that there are differing price structures for coffins and flowers; with 'The Last Supper' coffin tending to be the more expensive.

On the downside, one cannot book a private venue for the post-service refreshments (wake) because of the possibility that private venues could change their names, owners and/or price structures at a later date.

With pre-paid funerals, one gets to tailor one's own passage of way according to personal taste. This can include choosing one's favourite song to be played at the service and even instructions for the mourners (not necessarily to sob on cue, some don't want anybody to be there at all).

Then there is the purchasing of the grave, which can cost some £2,000. Then, if you cross districts, so you can be buried with your family members, you could pay up to £3,000 extra. This fee is payable because you are not paying council tax in the district you want to be buried in.

Last but not least and to finish the job off, bespoke gravestones can cost as much as £2,500. So perhaps a personally chosen, novel inscription etched onto the stone after you have departed this world is another valid reason to pre-pay for the arrangements.

Remembering of course that nagging doubt that some of the living relatives (only some) could (only could) be tempted to cut corners should they preside over the cost of your funeral. They could also keep you refrigerated and indefinitely delayed while they squabble over who pays what. There could then be a dilemma as to whether or not they can get the day off work to show up for your special event. It's worth keeping in mind though that the next of kin is not necessarily the living spouse or eldest sibling, it is the person (friend or family member) who has been most involved in your (the deceased person's) care.

The Real East-Enders

The Whitechapel district of East London has more to offer than meets the eye. We have the fascinating Krays' legend, the Elephant Man, and Jack the Ripper all in the same vicinity. The London Tourist Board needs to harness these potentially massive tourist attractions with immediate effect.

The Blind Beggar pub on the Whitechapel Road is the scene synonymous with the murder of George Cornell (originally known as George Myers) by Ronnie Kray on March 9th 1966. Although the layout of the pub is still the same today, the décor has obviously changed somewhat in comparison to the monochrome, but trendy, 1960s. A tourist attraction styled in the 1960s could be one way forward.

There were eleven murders committed in the Whitechapel locale between April 1888 and February 1891, with the infamous Jack the Ripper thought be responsible for five of them. Today, the guides taking the walking tour of the Whitechapel district can try too hard to be showmen-comedians, which is not to everyone's preference. For my part, I would prefer to be informed of the facts, as they occurred, with unknown titbits thrown in because of the inside information the guide would have previously researched. I personally deduced that the romanticised notion of the Ripper being a member of the royal family is rather incongruous. The person who committed the Whitechapel murders must have known the area very well to make their escape. The savage nature of the wounds inflicted on the victims (including prostitute Mary Kelly) suggests that the Ripper could have been a local butcher or something like.

Note: during the subsequent investigation with regard to the murder of Mary Kelly, a photograph was taken of her eyes, believing that those same eyes would contain an image of the last person she had seen.

Joseph (not John) Merrick was born in Leicester in 1862 and went to London with a touring freak show. He was in fact put into a shop window on the Whitechapel Road (now a sari shop) as a curiosity for people to stare at. A copy of his skeleton is exhibited in the Royal London Hospital, also on the Whitechapel Road. The film, *The Elephant Man* (1980), starring John Hurt, has to be one of the finest pictures ever produced. The part where he beseeches to the effect that he is not an elephant, not an animal, but a human being, is most poignant and soul-searches the toughest amongst us. The Elephant Man died in 1890 aged twenty-seven.

I would go as far to speculate that we have all felt like the Elephant Man at times.

Transporting Philosophy to Glastonbury

Having examined the academic on-line interpretations regarding the meaning of philosophy and when philosophical thinking is demonstrated, I drew a blank. My understanding of what philosophy is, appears to clash with that which is ascribed by our 'experts'.

I believe that a philosopher is someone who has views of the world/ humanity outside the parameters of convention and converses in such terms.

For example: *what would our world be and how would we make sense of it, had we not ascribed names for everything on it? What is that above one calls the sky? We ascribe it the name 'sky'; but what really is it?*

Or:

An insect the size of a pinhead refuses to crawl onto my hand when I box it in and coerce it to do so. This demonstrates that this living creature has a level of understanding.

Or:

What is time? Had not ancient dictatorships measured for how long they would colonise any given nation, there would probably be no such thing.

Another example of philosophy can sometimes have cynical connotations and can manifest into sayings or proverbs.

Many of us believe in the afterlife as a place of paradise; but not many of us are in a hurry to visit.

Famous historical philosophers like Aristotle advocated that the 'ladder of life' has eleven rungs, at the top of which are human beings. Not convinced on that one I'm afraid; especially when science informs that in the event of a cataclysmic occurrence, it would be cockroaches and rats that would undoubtedly survive, which points to the fact that we are not as resourceful as other creatures and so therefore cannot possibly be on the top rung of the ladder of life.

Anyhow, on a different vein, one does not have to be a philosopher to note that the train ride from London Paddington to Somerset (en route to Glastonbury) was the observed simile of riding in a heap of dilapidated scrap iron; our railway infrastructures are an international embarrassment.

Keeping with rails, what felt like a whistle-stop tour of Glastonbury, including the Abbey, and the famous Ancient Tor, was brief. And no, you don't have to wrestle with those youngsters in the mud to enjoy it. It did not take deep philosophical thinking either, to observe that accessibility to the Tor was limited for those who struggle with their mobility. It was at this point I had that light bulb moment stemming, of course, from deep philosophical genius: what about a simple cable car to scale the Tor so everybody can delight in it?

It was at the bus stop though, where I waited one hour and a half for a bus back to Taunton, that the most scholarly, philosophically discursive colloquy arose. The big talking point for locals was not 7th C Norman ruins, but the ruination of their bus service, which is being cut back to such a cruel extent, it is leaving many stranded and housebound.

Seems to be the national picture, doesn't it?

Wheel 'Em In

In 2012, Chris Grayling – who was Minister of State, Employment, Work and Pensions – together with the controversial private medical company Atos, were in the firing line again regarding ESA (the new replacement benefit for Income Support).

Even the mental health charity MIND pulled out of a review of its operations, calling the new guidelines for support 'inhumane'.

The new prerequisites for ESA payments at this time did not just penalise those with congenital diseases. Under the new scoring system, one got *nils* points (no points) for undergoing chemotherapy for cancer if it was not administered intravenously.

In fact the new ESA questionnaire was littered with more snares than a farmer's field, according to one adviser, which begs the question:

What have we come to?

It is thought that more than a thousand sickness benefit claimants died in 2011 after being told they were fit for work. The stress it is causing others who are repeatedly being called in for strict medical tests, for those appealing (costing millions) or for those having their benefits suspended indefinitely, cannot be quantified.

Those with serious physical and mental health problems are now having their benefits stopped for reasons such as: if one can stand or sit for longer than fifteen minutes, or they can both stand and sit in a cyclical scenario (a checkout operator in the new low-paid multinational 'superstore factory assembly lines', for example). Then again, has anybody else noticed how customers in or out of work now have to endure the duties that staff members used to endure? Self-checkout at supermarkets, reading your own electricity meter, the list is endless and is distressing for many. The multinationals have a 'little arrangement' going on, where customers are inadvertently working, or taking on extra duties, without even being aware of it.

Also in 2011, a supermarket in Westminster was forced to close because it was invaded by protesters angered by a job advert seeking permanent workers in exchange for expenses and jobseeker's allowance.

Although, during the Thatcher era, when shock and horror greeted the notion that the blind could put cherries on cakes, in the coalition era, even amputees were deemed fit to do a shift. Are disability groups therefore shooting themselves in the proverbial foot when maintaining that those in wheelchairs should not be treated any differently than the rest of us?

Some would argue they play right into governmental hands.

For those who cannot walk to the superstore factories; what do the multinational employers/government officials want to do?

Wheel 'em in?

On Queue for Salisbury, Southampton, Berkshire and South East London

Us British know our place, don't we, and my oh my, how we queue on order without question. We have no choice, whether it be at the post office to dutifully pay for the licensed privilege of watching BBC programming, or at theatres, checkouts, football grounds… the list is endless, and we do it all without a gripe. Well most of us do, anyway. When I was kid, and you were waiting for a while, you would shout "Shop", which was a customary vocal implement to attract the shopkeeper's attention. Not so sure it would have the same impact if shouted out while stuck in a long queue though – but when trapped in a queue for a long time, anything is worth a try.

After queuing for so long to buy my train ticket to Salisbury to see Stonehenge for the first time, I reasoned that fantasising/dolly daydreaming could help pass the time spent in the queue… On arrival in Salisbury railway station, a suspicious cloak and dagger-appearing character, peering over a copy of the *Mail*, sat opposite me. I spy with my little eye something beginning with F, one mused: Fabrication, Fake, Feigned, Footle, False, Fantasy. Can anyone else think of more appropriate F words for the recent nerve agent poisonings in the city? Answers on a postcard, please, and no swear-words.

When finding myself on the grounds of Salisbury Cathedral (not on queue) it was a little disappointing that a troupe of green space suit-wearing conspiracy theory aficionados, complete with black bluebottle-like gas masks, did not surface, headed by our poison-tongued foreign secretary supremo, Batty Boris, also sporting matching turquoise wellies. Instead, a fairy tale setting to depict the modern Russian Ogre fairy tale, set the fabled panorama (yes, two more F words there).

There wasn't a sinner in sight.

Stonehenge was next on the agenda. It seemed impossible to make your own way to Amesbury, where the ancient stones are in situ, although I did bear witness to a car park when I arrived. You had to pay £15 for the bus journey and that was that. When dutifully paying my fare (after queuing of course) I thought, well, £15 to visit the world-famous neolithic site was not that expensive, only for the bus driver to inform me that you also had to pay up to £20 on top of the £15 for one's entrance fee.

£35 to visit Stonehenge is excessive just to look at a pile of old bricks and a few old barns (yes, some would argue that this vulgar statement could only be made by the non-educated and cultureless amongst us). This is not the case. It's because I understand the importance of historical education, in that the masses would struggle to pay such a disproportionate entrance fee, that the crass utterance was made. It was observed just before entering (after queuing again) that the kiosk operator had me hold on for two minutes while he rolled up a massive wad of twenties to place them in a blue tube to send on to English Heritage (or better still, to some director's back pocket). 1.3 million visitors a year: add that up into pounds, shillings and pence.

There were also queues for the shuttle up to the Stoney location, so I just bit my stiff upper-lip, and got on with it. What is more, when arriving at the circle, one did so in queues of sorts, a queue with an extra-large Japanese contingent, might I add. Perhaps £35 is not a great deal in yen.

When I did catch site (yes, I know I have mis sighted) of the gigantic boulders for the first time, it did appear like something out of a film. Nevertheless, hordes of French kids getting in the way soon brought one back to real life with a crash. It wasn't a pleasant experience, immersed with the tourist types, enacting their rehearsed smiles and poses to declare superior cultural quintessence on Facebook.

Personally, I never really bought the idea that the stones were hauled over from South Wales or nearby Marlborough; well, why would our ancient folk endure such physical torture even within the realms of the slave-driven scheme of things. We weren't as daft as the Romans and Anglo Saxons like to paint us, you know. Although the real facts of the mystery may never be unearthed, I would go along with the recent idea that the stones have always been there, which is why they were deemed so important to our ancient ancestors.

One could say that the bus ride on the double-decker back to Salisbury (April, 2018) was a little more interesting. No, one is not referring to the ancient burial mounds on show at Old Sarum (where maybe another payment and a little more queueing would be on the cards – I didn't fall for that one). Having not checked into my hotel yet, and unsure how to find it (the bus for Stonehenge had left from the railway station), I spotted my bed for the night (hotel) as we pulled into the town and so naturally pressed the bell to get off. Subsequently, I was admonished by the disgruntled bus driver in that I could not get off the bus and would have to sit back down and wait for the designated stop. Yes, sort of on queue; yours truly reluctantly obeyed. To the disdain of fellow passengers, I declared to the bus driver that they could not force passengers to remain on the bus. Rebel rousing aside, the Grenfell Tower sprang to mind as I watched my hotel disappear into a strange and confused architectural horizon, in that officials tell us to stay put at all costs for our own safety. They've got no chance, thank you very much. If I deemed any space even slightly perilous, my gut instinct would be to escape any possible would-be spatial entombing.

Apart from Wiltshire, the next stop on my tour would be a landmark in Hampshire which I had always wanted to visit. Always being Southampton-curious, the Titanic Museum informed me that many in the city knew someone who had perished in the 1912 disaster. At the museum, an inquiry was depicted to determine if third class passengers were barred from exiting onto the deck when the ship was going down. It was found that they were not. Some people can tell bare-faced lies on oath, you know.

On the way home from Southampton, the train was halted in Reading (Berkshire) due to signal problems at Oxford. We were then informed by the train manager that even the trains were stuck in a queue. Due in South East London for the Millwall vs Bristol City game the very next day, and after examining alternative routes via Swindon, I headed for nearby Slough to stay overnight instead. This would be a life-changing experience, in that I would experience first-hand what it feels like to be in an ethnic minority in a multiracial city.

Still, nearby Windsor Castle was recommended by the hotel manager, so I decided to visit the very next day: Not being a royalist myself, it was still an interesting excursion, especially when a modern-day, or Tudor-like, king's assassin-come-armed police officer, patrolled the surrounding streets for the Changing of the Guard ceremony. I could see it in the face of one such uniformed officer. He could kill. Talking of Windsor, did you know that for Harry and Megs' wedding in May 2018, those who reside in Windsor could let their homes out for up to £3,500 per night? Any takers?

My first Millwall game was my next port of call, having recently adopted them as one of my top teams (having always been attracted to the underdog; maybe because I'm an underdog myself). That aside, I was unaware that this particular game would afford me one of those rare silent chuckles the more cynical amongst us seldom experience. I don't know if it was imagined or not, but when the ball went out of play, a Lions fan threw it back to the Bristol City player on the touch line with such velocity I thought it was going to knock the player over; talk about the extra man.

It also has to be recorded that before the match in question had kicked off, I and countless others had formed a long orderly queue to collect our tickets, paid for online. At about 14.30, one young fan vacated the queue (but left his mate holding his place). He returned a few minutes later to tell all within earshot that if you go to the main ticket counter (where you pay for match tickets on the day) which was queue-less, and state that you have already collected your prepaid ticket/s but have lost them, they will issue your ticket/s again straight away, thus avoiding the soul-destroying lengthy column of human bodies.

Deliberating on whether to become very un-British in order to get out of the queueing mire, saw me waiting until around 14.50 to ask a man standing next to me to hold my place while I went on a reconnaissance mission to estimate the distance from the front of the queue to where we were standing. When I got to the front of that queue, it was determined that I would probably enter the Den as late as 15.30 if I obediently remained standing in the queue awaiting my turn. The decision was then made to 'blag it', so a tale about losing my ticket was told at the alternative tickets on the day counter.

For my yarn-spinning endeavours my ticket was printed out there and then.

On returning to the queue flashing my shiny new ticket, I informed others around that perhaps it was expected that fans would tell a little white lie, so they would not miss out on an event they had paid up-front for.

As I navigated my way to Cold Blow Lane, I didn't turn back to see if those others were still waiting in the queue.

Perhaps they are still there.

A Long Way from Tipperary to Newcastle for Sister Agnes

It was while out canvassing for votes in the May 2014 local elections that I bumped into my former deputy headmistress, Sister Agnes, at the Convent of Mercy on London Road, Newcastle-under-Lyme. I was a pupil in her class in 1973. The school in question was St Peters in Cobridge, Stoke-on-Trent. I have fond memories of the three no-nonsense nuns who presided over St Peters (or Cobridge RC) in those years, namely Sister Agnes, Sister Philomena and the headmistress of the day, Sister Gerard.

Some things one never forgets. It was in Sister Agnes's top class that I was beaten into second place during a spelling test for spelling the word carol 'caroll'. Yes, I was devastated. Although, if the same had occurred today, I would have argued the toss and made the argument that technically my spelling was also correct (Lewis Carroll, for example). Additionally, it was after a school trip to a country house as an eleven-year-old writing a follow-up story that Sister Agnes taught me how to grapple with the tricky concepts surrounding tenses and time referents.

Referents apart, education is forever ongoing because it was at the Convent of Mercy on London Road, Newcastle-under-Lyme where I would learn about the retreat called 'Coolock' and the history of the Sisters of Mercy in Newcastle-under-Lyme.

Historically, the first community of the Sisters of Mercy was established in the Holy Trinity parish when Mother Bernard left Scotland and founded the convent in 1892. The beautiful stained glass windows in the adjoining chapel were later imported from Dublin.

Sister Agnes, now eighty-five, entered the order at sixteen as a postulant. Originally from County Tipperary in Ireland, it was her then teacher Sister Philomena, on leave from the convent in Newcastle-under-Lyme, who inspired Mary Burke (as she was then known) to become a nun herself. The year was 1949.

Sister Agnes would then undergo vocational teacher training in Liverpool from 1951–53, and from 1955–59 she would teach at St Mary's Junior School in Stanier Street, Newcastle. More importantly, it was when she taught at St Peters in Cobridge in the years 1959–83 that I became acquainted with her. She retired from the school in 1983, aged fifty.

After reminiscing about people and places gone by, Sister Agnes (still exuding that same shrewd sangfroid as she did all those years ago) showed me the class register of 1973 and then disclosed proudly, in her soft Tipperary accent:

"I have the names and register of every pupil in every class I have ever taught but I have been retired for a while now."

When I pressed more regarding the history of the convent, Sister Agnes said:

"The convent used to be a hat makers' home and was originally a Georgian building and school. The nuns initially relied on the generosity of local people to become established. In 1926 there also used to be a 'Poor Man's Porch' at the entrance to the convent."

Keeping the Wolves at Bay

It makes a refreshing change when a public figure, like a police chief constable, holds up his hands and admits mistakes were made (in this case the errors made policing the Port Vale v Wolverhampton Wanderers fixture in 2013).

This enables sensible and transparent dialogue to ensue with all parties, which ensures the same miscalculations are not made again. In contrast, when the shutters go down and institutions refuse point blank to accept their part in any wrongdoing, it only fuels suspicion and resentment for those aggrieved, where a long and protracted complaints process can result.

There were some questions that needed answering regarding the aftermath of Port Vale's match against Wolverhampton Wanderers. It was not just about police actions, but about the lupine policy of unleashing police dogs during a potential violent fracas per se; which can result in the deep and ugly bite wounds as seen on the innocent few.

Even when walking down the street in one's own locality, it can fill one with dread when passing German Shepherd dogs (who are thought to be direct descendants of wolves). This wariness is exaggerated by the knowledge that perhaps the animals can sense your fear. Talking of which, although dogs could be used as a deterrent, some would argue that to actually unleash a dog (or wolf) on people in any circumstances (whether legally or illegally) is a barbarous act. Notwithstanding, to meet fear by using fear can only result in one thing – fear on both sides.

This is the unacceptable face of policing.

There are, no doubt, fair, decent and professional police officers out there who instil in us a sense of security. Equally, there are also those in the vein of the old-school thinking (even at a high level) who believe in the doctrine of containing/managing crime and disorder by force and at the expense of public confidence.

The Billion Pound Babble

The *Leaders' Debate* televised by ITV on April 2nd 2015 threw out some interesting differentials for the following general election of May 7th 2015. A rainbow of colours were now inclusive in the political process, instead of the usual boring and predictable greys of Conservative, Labour and Lib Dems respectively.

In saying that it was the same old same mould in many respects; during the two-hour debacle every one of the seven party leaders consistently spun the words millions, billions and even trillions of pounds to back up their arguments. In fact, every other sentence seemed to be punctuated with figures and stats, with the word billion uttered so many times it ceased to be believable.

Do you think these politicians are just quoting their own lucky numbers and then adding the word billion as an addendum? The billions babble has now become so virulent it is being paraphrased by every section of the media, which in turn has not become conducive to restoring faith in the politically apathetic. In my estimation, whoever concocts this baffling and annoying numerical spin needs putting under critical spotlight themselves.

Billions aside, from left to right and first in the firing line we had Natalie Bennett of the Green Party, who did make some convincing social arguments. The Green Party, however, always manages to let themselves down by over-liberalising (with loose immigration policies in this instance).

Next in line we had that impostor Nick Clegg of the Liberal Democrats, who just loves bleating billions too. As false as ever, it was fitting that every time he spoke, I fast-forwarded the recording. This is probably the choice the electorate will make on May 7th, as in not bother to listen to a word he says. We know what the Tories are; they say so on the tin. Before the last general election though, the Lib Dems labelled themselves as something quite different.

Third from left stood Nigel Farage of UKIP. In one episode not long into the show it seemed like 'all the fun at the fair' as he started to bobble (not babble) up and down like one of those laughing policemen. Farage also repeated himself over the national debt, in that Britain had allowed the peoples of ten (no, not ten billion) former communist countries to enter the country. He expanded on this point advocating that it was okay for French, Dutch and German immigrants to flow into our country but not for other Europeans to follow suit. How divisive is that?

Then we had Edward Samuel Miliband (Labour Party). Carefully choreographed, he reminded of a cheap B-movie actor as he manipulated the camera, complete with staged voice, which was over softly contrived to sound convincing (even when he threw in a billion or two stats for us to number crunch on). I don't know about anybody else, but I couldn't wait for the Labour Party to be decimated in Scotland. The so-called party of the people had it coming, didn't it?

Leanne Wood of Plaid Cymru stood centre right in the panel formation, although politically speaking she is anything but. Ms Wood did display that there is still fire in the Welsh dragon's belly as she elaborated on policy with cool and calming tones. Still, she did slip up with the B word once or twice. Although the desire for independence in Wales is currently near dormant, Welsh Nationalists can take heart from the fact that so was the desire for Scottish independence just a few years ago.

Second to last, but not least in the political spectrum, Nicola Sturgeon and the SNP had made this general election the most interesting contest in years. Although the SNP leader billionised her rhetoric too, she exuded a definite honesty. Not expounding on the authoritrian nature of the Europe the SNP want Scotland to be part of could cost some votes. Even so, the prospect of some kind of Labour/SNP coalition would've most definitely set the cat amongst the pigeons at Westminster.

Firmly on the far right of our screens stood David Cameron (Conservative). Dave, give me the number of your stylist so I can give them a good telling off. The bags under your eyes were showing, you know, (a little concealer could have put paid to that). In any event, it's no wonder you can't sleep at night with the misery you and your party are currently inflicting on the general populace. Also, on the right side of your bonce, your hair stuck out rather; a little like the mad professor. Yes, Dave, you would have to be stark raving bonkers to believe that your scatter-brained austerity argument will gain any further credence. How many billion will your rich chums stand to profit from those austere measures again?

As with Miliband and Clegg (the three identical triplets), Cameron used that old chestnut of responding to the author of the question (a member of the audience) by their first name (Johnny in one example) as if to generate affability with the questioner – a ruse probably learnt at some cheap political stage school in Eton.

In conclusion, I did not need a leaders' debate to help me decide who to vote for; yours truly was always going to vote for the SNP or Plaid Cymru. Hold on though, unlike my Scottish and Welsh counterparts who can vote for Labour, the Tories and the Lib Dems, here in England I cannot vote for the Scottish or Welsh assemblies.

I would therefore have to vote for the Green Party. Hmm… how many billion (in real terms of course) did they propose to spend on the NHS?

Some would espouse that, due to the inclusion of the smaller parties in the political process, politics in Britain has changed for the better; political dogma, however, (like the billions spin) appears to go unchecked.

King Herbert of Staffordshire

I have thought of a good stunt to get the tourists flocking to North Staffordshire. What's more, it would take the focus away from austerity and savage cuts to public services. Yes, we could unveil King Herbert of Staffordshire; who is to know he never existed a long, long, long, time ago?

It is beyond reasonable doubt that he could have been on the throne before the Anglo-Saxon invasion; a sort of fiery puddled type who was kind to his subjects but ruled with an iron fist.

His Majesty could have even had a hand in 'The Battle of Boslem'.

One would imagine that King Herbert was renowned for his royal oratories, possibly quoted in the *Doomsday Book*. Perhaps one memorable exclamation was something very regal, like:

"Dunner start me duck."

According to Reuters, "It was a warm day but I suddenly felt cold," was how Philippa Langley described the powerful sensation she experienced when she walked over the unmarked grave of her hero, King Richard III of England, buried beneath a social services car park in Leicestershire.

Perhaps we should check out Sainsbury's car park in Newcastle and see how many of us 'feel a chill' in any given spot. Who knows; it could be our very own King Herbert beneath our feet.

Key to Unlocking
Dementia Progression

In modern Britain people are living longer. However, it is thought that dementia affects up to 800,000 people in Great Britain, with 25 million of that population having a close friend or relative who suffers from the condition (2018). Coupled with the personal cost, dementia is a strain on the British economy to the tune of some £23 billion a year and, despite these figures, funds for research into Alzheimer's disease (the most common form of dementia) is at a minimum.

Dementia affects the short-term memory, where sufferers can forget what day it is. But to delve deeper with greater critical analysis one can disinter some interesting theories surrounding this progressive and debilitating condition. As the brain slows down with age, could those suffering from early-onset dementia be remembering only the most important aspects to their lives and discarding the rest?

At this point, perhaps we should magnify the fine line between old age forgetfulness and the beginning of early-onset dementia (formerly known as senile dementia). At the age of fifty-plus, many people start to forget details such as, for what reason did they enter a certain room, did they apply deodorant, or did they lock the back door? This memory loss can then progress to not knowing what day it is, what they did the day before, forgetting a conversational punch line mid-sentence, or even being unable to recall a close relative's Christian name. As we grow older our brains do too, so to mentally process life's demands, our memories can begin to stammer. The brain is a strange and unknown scientific terrain; some people experiencing memory problems can write up full meetings hours after the event with a high degree of accuracy but can't remember if they have brushed their teeth or not.

One hypothesis is that the brain is separating the important from the unimportant. For example, if a person is now retired, the need to remember the current day or what they did the day before, is way down the list of priorities of things to remember. Whereas when that person was in full-time work it was a necessity to be aware of what day it was and what their schedule would have been the previous day.

This suggests that with the onset of dementia comes self-imposed regulation of the essential things to remember while discarding the non-essential.

So in effect, could one successfully argue that the mind is in fact becoming stronger not weaker so that it can survive long-term?

The same can be said for those little indiscretions like forgetting to apply deodorant, perfume or after shave. By using your sense of smell to check if you applied them are you making this matter inconsequential and so resting your brain to remember the more significant events?

Although dementia is a cruel disease there are some compensations for being affected by it. Some sufferers at times believe they are younger or in their family environment in an era when they were safe and secure. Others are not aware of distressing events or even deaths in their own family and are not aware of their own predicament and possible early demise because of the disease.

It is thought that dementia sufferers have fleeting moments of lucidity that last for seconds and it is unknown whether or not they understand conversations around them fleetingly or not. Routine and distractions are also pivotal in any discursive analysis around the subject of early-onset dementia.

Almost like a contradiction in terms, it is vital for those suffering from dementia to break the routine of the day by undertaking activities that stretch the mind from the ongoing monotony. This can take the shape of a walk outside or participating in an activity group or game including browsing old photographs, preferably in the company of a living relative. This will, by all accounts, allow the dementia sufferer's brain to become less idle, as the brain will be embracing different undertakings to deal with in any given day. Yes, work it.

In conclusion, we must ask the question when does early-onset dementia become Alzheimer's disease? Could it be equated to the same metaphor when distinguishing the difference between forgetting to lock the back door and putting the back door key in the freezer compartment?

I Would Harm a Fly

I have always had a thing about houseflies. They are grotesque. Even as a kid, if one flew into our house, first size would be ascertained. This meant that if the fly was a bluebottle I would cry, "Big Bugger". This was a cue to reach for the tennis rackets and if you hit a bluebottle mid-air with the racket, you would hear a pinging sound from the racket strings connecting with the insect, which was a direct hit and could slice the fly in two at the thorax. Yellow matter would then ooze out of its cadaver.

It can also be brought to mind when a fly started to act in a strange insane way after being discovered in my bedroom during the winter months (note the pesky pests are not usually active in winter). Instead of flying off to avoid me, it was so disorientated it sort of went for me which elicited wild screams on my part.

Talking of which, as a twenty-three-year-old putting the rubbish out, I can reminisce shrieking like a nine-year-old girl. As the dustbin lid was lifted, I was met with a chicken carcass discarded a few days before; it was now riddled with maggots.

Keeping with the screaming theme, one lady described how she could not get her teenage son to clean his room and so leftover foodstuffs remained on his plate, in his room, for days. Then, one night, a piercing squeal emanated from the upstairs room, to which a thundering hoofing boom could be heard descending the stairs. The teenager then plonked down his decayed morsels that were by now teeming with maggots. He then ran back upstairs. As the story goes, mother's darker cruel side then surfaced as instead of immediately disposing of the wrigglers hygienically, she immersed them in bleach as some sort of cleansing ritual.

Scientifically speaking, diseases carried by house flies include salmonella, anthrax, tuberculosis, typhoid, cholera and dysentery. In saying that, if the flying invader gains entry into my home, firstly, I leave the window open to give them a chance to vamoose before resorting to giving them a good gassing with the fly spray.

I don't want to dispose of their dirty corpses, you see.

Not only can they smell death from four miles away and are attracted to dog faeces and anything decomposing, flies will vomit and excrete onto your food to then suck it back in through their proboscis, which is a plunger-like attachment that extends from the bottom of the head. They then regurgitate the lethal mix back onto your food.

Houseflies have impeccable table manners, you know.

And to think, some people act very nonchalantly or pretend that they have not seen the flies if they are buzzing around their home or in a café where they are working. I have borne witness to that benign wafting or shooing enaction, to demonstrate to others that yes, they have clocked the blighter. Equally, some restaurant staff can't be bothered to play-act. In November 2018, I visited an up-market restaurant in town and after being seated in a plush, discreet table by the window, I was informed that there was a fly behind me. Expecting a small fruit fly or something similar, I was a little concerned to be confronted with a large bluebottle. Now not content with dining at the eatery and feeling a little queasy, I raised the fly issue with a staff member who then equipped himself with a rolled-up cloth napkin. He then flick-whipped the insect and killed it just as another big bluebottle appeared in the same area. When he proceeded to remove the dead bluebottle from the scene, another one appeared, so in effect, I had seen three large size bluebottles in a small area in the space of eight minutes. After bearing witness to the third insect I was propelled toward the exit and out of the door – never to return again may I add.

Let's be thankful the staff member did not pick up the dead insect with his hands, when imagining that some people can handle flies in order to pull off their wings makes me physically heave. I would have to use a microscope if I ever had to examine a bluebottle close-up. Have you not yet been acquainted with those large beady eyes?

It goes without saying that Bluebottles or flies are associated with all things grisly as their habits suggest. In saying the above, there could be seen a fly confliction in the excellent movie Psycho (1960). When Norman Bates, played expertly by Anthony Perkins (in mother mode), states that he/she wouldn't harm a fly in reference to the pretence that he (or she) was not guilty of the murders, the statement denoted the fly as innocent.

Not the case I'm afraid.

Going to Toon

I don't know about Catherine Cookson, but I believe I can tell the Geordies a good tale me sel. Hard fact is stranger than fiction and sometimes the general populace can be uncomfortable hearing those cold hard personal home truths.

So let's convey those less harsh facts; they might not be as juicy, but interesting all the same. Not forgetting that our use of factual language is governed by our own self-imposed censorship. And of course the audience we write for dictates that censorship.

Having always been interested in Newcastle-upon-Tyne for some years, it took quite a while to actually visit the now modern metropolis set in Tyne and Wear (Newcastle used to be in Northumberland). Initially, when I first exited the railway station, Newcastle was nothing like what I expected. Subsequently, I was taken aback by how sophisticated the city of Newcastle and its people were/are.

One drawback was the price of the hotels in Newcastle and Gateshead, which can be very expensive, to say the least. One can pay some £85 for a room per night. What I and many others found annoying about such sky-high prices was that it was nearly a tenner for your breakfast to boot (which amounted to near on £100 per night for hotel room and breakfast in a central location).

Another surprise when visiting Newcastle was that if you take a stroll down to the Quayside you will find yourself in Gateshead; it appears that the two are connected by the north and south banks of the River Tyne.

Quays aside, a trip to St James' Park, which is very centrally located, is well worth penning onto your to do list when visiting Newcastle. Tickets for lesser band games can be purchased online for as little as £27.

Although Newcastle has many points of interest, for me it was the attraction of the people and their original vernacular that focalises the point. Words like 'pet' are used when addressing you personally, which can be endearing to the independent vacationer. Furthermore, 'Geordies' (the word Geordie probably originated from local miners in the North-East who used the word to describe safety lamps designed by George Stephenson in 1815, not from those Geordie Jeans clothes shops of the 1980s) seem to have an original manner in relating and expressing themselves, not just to outsiders but to each other. Is this the most important generic factor that strikes visitors when they land on the banks of Newcastle-on-Tyne and Gateshead for the first time?

Why aye man (of course it is).

Inside O'Connor Part 1: Prelude to Pre-rehabilitation

Alcohol is a causal factor in scores of medical conditions, including cancer, cirrhosis of the liver, and depression

Liver disease through alcohol abuse is prevalent in young people today in a way that was not seen some thirty years ago. It is thought that alcohol problems affect ten million people in Britain and the British are the heaviest boozers in Europe. Furthermore, tens of thousands die every year through alcohol abuse and even more die from associated diseases caused by alcohol. To say nothing of the 17 million working days lost per year through alcohol misuse the night before. The negative effect alcohol also has on domestic family life and society in general is incalculable.

As alcohol dependency and drug abuse grows nationwide, so does the number of people who need more specialised help and support. The BAC O'Connor Centre in Clayton Road, Newcastle-under-Lyme, Staffordshire, provided that support. Opened in 1998, the O'Connor gained numerous awards including a Healthcare Commission score of excellent – the highest in the country.

Being lucky enough to be given the chance to research the workings of the O'Connor Centre in depth, from the inside out, over a two-month period, has enabled this series to be relayed with some accuracy. I once thought that an addict was a term used for a heroin or crack cocaine addict. The word addict is commonly used in rehab and throughout this series as terminology to describe those suffering with addiction issues.

It also has to be said that there was another wing of the O'Connor Centre in Burton-on-Trent, which offered the same facility but with extras, like resident doctors and medical staff. This is the ideal solution if a couple are both substance abusers, in that they would not be allowed to enter the same rehabilitation centre together. They would be split up; one would go to Burton and one to Newcastle.

Note: if a couple both have addiction issues, for one to become clean and the other to remain in addiction is not a recipe for success for either.

With regard to alcohol, if one is ready to stop consuming there are some things one ought to know, the most important of which is, do not just stop if you are drinking heavily. You need to see your doctor for advice where you could be referred to hospital for detoxification, or 'detox'. In hospital you can be treated before you enter rehabilitation.

Addictions are not just alcohol-based. One can be addicted to opiates (including heroin), cannabis and even prescription drugs. Whatever one's poison, many residents who entered the O'Connor Centre were at the juncture of a life and death situation. There were also those residents who had been binge drinking most nights, or using drugs recreationally, and on the precipice of full-blown addiction. This is how endemic the situation is; those predisposed will always progress into the inevitable fall of drug/drink-addled mayhem.

After first seeing their doctor for substance abuse issues, addicts would be referred to a social worker. Rehab was not just a preserve of the rich and famous. The social worker would then apply for funding from the local authority, which can cost in excess of £500 per week for a stay at the O'Connor Centre. The programme in rehab would last for some four months.

If residents were claiming ESA before they entered rehab they would carry on being in receipt of it. The same applied to housing benefit. Residents would also be charged some £25 (2011) towards the cost of their stay including meals, which they would pay into the office. Some residents leave the O'Connor owing rent.

If one decides to enter rehab, it was best policy to turn up at the O'Connor in Clayton Road for an informal pre-rehab group meeting on a Thursday afternoon at 1pm. Here, other people with substance abuse problems would be present, some under the influence.

It must be said that one would have to push one's case to the duty staff member at pre-rehab to secure a place at the centre if one were serious about coming off substances. A current resident of the O'Connor Centre can also co-chair the meeting with the staff member on duty. This enables those present to ask any questions they see fit. Most questions revolve around the permission to have one's mobile phone during the stay – one could not. Other questions include visiting times – which were/are for a couple of hours a week on a Saturday morning.

A special visit in the week was available in exceptional circumstances, which had to be granted by a therapist. Another frequent question was if one can access TV on a regular basis. TV was limited to two hours a night and on special occasions.

Visits were not allowed for any resident during the first few weeks and once one was allowed visitors that visitor could take the resident away from the compound for the duration of the visit if they chose.

Day care was also an option. On day care, residents engage with the O'Connor during working hours some five days a week and Saturday mornings. In other words, they do not live in, can keep their mobile phones and they go home on an evening. Technically, for the fatuous and those predisposed to cheating, this can allow one to drink (or to take some drugs that do not stay long in the system) on a Saturday evening. Then they will not have to supply a breath test on Sunday and so can then pass the breath test on the Monday morning (whenever a resident exits, then re-enters the building they will always be breathalysed).

At this point it must be said that some entering rehab were doing so due to a court order or to regain custody of their children. Elements within this category sometimes devised ingenious methods in order to smuggle drugs into the centre.

Inside O'Connor Part 2: The Dignified Strip

Antidepressant items prescribed and dispensed by physicians in England has more than doubled in the last twenty years

When one has gained the all clear from the doctor at the Burton-on-Trent BAC, the O'Connor Centre, the new resident is given a date for admittance. With cases packed, the prospective resident has to pass the breathalyser in the office foremost to show they are 'clean'. Many forms have to be signed at this time which can take up to two or three hours. All medication (including antidepressants) is taken from the resident and only medication that is absolutely necessary is allowed. This is construed as a positive policy as so many people rely on prescription drugs that are not really necessary. It becomes difficult to access an aspirin for a headache once being admitted to the BAC in Newcastle. However, although this policy was live in 2011, in 2012 taking antidepressants by residents was allowed.

Then comes the strip search, which by all accounts is a dignified process as in one wears a paper gown. There is no internal. The search is a necessary prerequisite because addicts have smuggled all sorts in with them in the past. Antiperspirant spray is also confiscated, as are razor blades. Yes, those desperate enough have been known to drink antiperspirant or aftershave in the hope that the alcohol content in the solutions will intoxicate them. Your bag is then taken up to your room by a staff member because the landings where your room is located will be locked in the day time. There are separate male and female wings and it is forbidden to cross-visit the landings.

One is then taken into the main lounge area where other residents may be sitting, although at this time, most of the residents could be in therapy or doing other things like sorting out utility bills with a staff member. In fact, all the worries of bills, rent and debts will be dealt with by an in-house staff member, the majority of whom are ex-addicts themselves. Many addicts prior to admittance to the O'Connor have been severely isolated or living a dangerous life. Some might even be ex-prisoners. Others are teachers, manual workers, nurses, prison officers and even ex-police officers. Addiction does not discriminate.

You are then assigned your own therapist and will partake in group therapy and workshops most days. There are also holistic therapies like massage and the therapy of whale sounds and acupuncture.

The residents soon become drawn to certain therapists and different therapy suits different needs. Some would argue that certain aspects of the therapy are questionable, as in the 'humiliation therapy', for want of a better term. Comments by one resident to another in a group scenario of, "You don't look safe in your own skin", have been heard to be voiced. Other questionable lines of therapy can be seen when a therapist puts another person down to make the person undergoing the therapy feel better. This is a controversial means of therapy which some argue is counterproductive, as in, you may make one person feel better by comparing them to another in the same group room, but this could be at the expense of the person being put down.

One soon realises that there are continual key words used throughout the process of rehab which are quickly mimicked by the residents, such as 'projection', 'grounded', 'group', 'aftercare', 'grateful' and 'in a nice place'. There is also the rescuing theory where if a resident defends a person being verbally attacked in 'group' (group therapy) it would be frowned upon. It is believed that the one being verbally attacked should learn to fend for themselves which would apparently empower that same person.

Many residents exclaimed that their one-on-one therapy (just the resident and the therapist) was beneficial to their mental state. One supposes that not so many people had been interested in the addict when they were in the dark and lonely place of addiction. There are differing types of therapists, all with differing ideas. One therapist went out of their way to try and incite a resident to cry, perhaps believing a good sob would unburden them. Another therapist could be quite intimidating at times and exploited personality foibles (for what benefit is anyone's guess). By and large though, most of the therapists were good decent people who cared about others.

The age group of residents varied, but there did seem to be a greater number of residents in their forties. There were those in their twenties, thirties, fifties and even sixties, it has to be said. The alcohol intake for the majority before admittance was astounding; litres of spirits were drunk on sittings or 'sprees'. During this time the addict would not eat, wash or even rouse from the sofa. A significant section of the residents were on the brink of death before they made the decision to come into the O'Connor. The same could be said for the heroin addicts, where tales of robbing their mother's jewellery to fund their addiction surfaced during group.

Inside O'Connor Part 3: The Strange Incantation

It can be argued that if those addicted to substances were offered the choice to sign for compulsory rehab (they cannot discharge for the duration) instead of jail terms, they would do so willingly. With the end result being a safer and more empowered community

It costs the NHS over two billion per year to treat alcohol and opiate-related incidents, with the overall cost rising substantially when adding up the total expenditure on the criminal justice system. Therefore, isn't it simple logic to treat addiction before it progresses to incarceration? It is thought that as a nation, we spend up to £40,000 per year, per prisoner (2018).

The BAC O'Connor Centre, in Newcastle-under-Lyme, was slightly less expensive than other rehabs in the country. It is also true to say that those addicts with means have a better chance of survival than those who do not; but that survival intrinsically depends on the individual, as in the addict must want to change their lives if they are to succeed. Some argue that rehab programmes are brainwashing of sorts. If they are, then it could be described as a positive brainwashing, because the addict's life has been so chaotic; many have to go back to basics to learn the fundamentals of healthy living again.

The word 'process' cropped up at the BAC Newcastle often. It is where the resident group at the rehab centre meet to start the day. Having been checked at hourly intervals during the night the resident will be called at 7.30am to get up, having spent the first night in their new room. The rooms were pretty basic but clean and fresh and residents soon begin to adorn them with their own regalia (mostly family photographs).

The meals were average but above average, or even gourmet, for those used to a liquid or narcotic dinner. Breakfast was usually cereal and toast, lunch (or dinner) consisted of soup and a ham salad baguette, and dinner (or tea for some) was a meal of fish or meat, potatoes and veg with a dessert.

During the first week new arrivals will not be allocated a menial household task to complete in the daytime, but they will still engage in Process. Process is called at approximately 9.30am, where residents sit in a circle and are breathalysed one by one (one blows through a plastic tube into a black box held by the house staff member present). There will be a captain of the group who will go around every individual present and ask them how they are feeling. The captain system is worked out on the fact that the last person to enter rehab will be the last person to take captaincy and so on until the resident works their way up the pecking order after a couple of months to become first vice-captain, then captain.

Rehab is a revolving door where someone is always due to 'graduate' (an event when the resident has successfully completed the programme which will be elaborated on at a later interval) and another resident is being booked in.

It is during Process that key words like 'grateful" and such-like begin to emerge. After everyone says their piece, the captain asks if there are any house issues and turns to the staff member to ask if there are any staff issues. It is then that an enactment (which can be strange to some) occurs. Everyone attending, stands up, joins hands in a circle and says the Serenity Prayer. This prayer is said at AA and NA meetings and is an American concept based on the steps one has to take to be drug/alcohol free.

Some argue that it is quasi-religious. Others argue that it is not. When one resident asked another resident why they joined in the circle, held hands but would not say the prayer, the resident replied that they would feel ridiculous to do so. There are many versions of the prayer but the one used at rehab does not use the word God: It goes something like this:

"Grant me the serenity
To accept the things I cannot change.
The courage to change the things I can
And the wisdom to know the difference."

The circle of people then swing their arms out, holding the next person's hand, while saying a sort of encore. Then everyone gently squeezes the hand of the person they are holding hands with. Some of the new residents are shocked by this enactment, but it seems to uplift the more seasoned. After this ritual the residents then go to the rota to check where they are for what group and with what therapist. Process and the ritual just described is repeated at approximately 9pm that same day. Then there are two hours to watch TV, play pool or table tennis, read, or write up their 'Feelings Diary'. This diary is a written record penned by the resident of how they were feeling that day. Residents are not encouraged to stay up after midnight.

There was also an option for residents to join a local gym or leisure centre during their time at the BAC, which they are encouraged to visit once or twice a week. Ingrained defective behaviours can surface during gym enrolment, where some residents would try to 'sneak in' without paying.

Inside O'Connor Part 4: Smokers' Corner in Big Bro

Smoking causes numerous death related illnesses including lung cancer, emphysema, strokes, and heart disease

There are various statistics including guestimates on how many addicts are actually successful in keeping off drugs (including alcohol) after going through a programme of rehabilitation. The BAC O'Connor Centre in Newcastle-under-Lyme offered a very short programme compared to other rehabs internationally. This does not mean that the O'Connor is any less successful. Accurate data is hard to come by on those that relapse or lapse, mainly because those relapsing are sometimes loath to admit that they are using again. Educated estimates point to the possibility that three out of twenty addicts who enter rehab successfully stay off drugs indefinitely.

Believe it or not, this is a good result.

The addict, on completing the programme, can sometimes use their favoured drug less or swap one drug for another (cross addiction). Some ex-heroin users can then use cannabis or alcohol as a replacement on quitting; kidding themselves they have chosen the lesser of the two evils. Or they use their original drug of choice more intermittently; but this almost inevitably leads back to full-blown addiction.

To be successful in overcoming addiction one has to come off all drugs, period. Even tobacco, one might ask? Disease due to smoking kills more people per annum than drugs, although death is not directly imminent through smoking. It is most odd, then, that approximately 80% of residents at the O'Connor smoke and head straight for Smokers' Corner after group. What next; a rehab for smokers?

At the BAC O'Connor Centre, overt personal relationships with another resident were not tolerated. If two residents became over friendly they would be warned first and, if they persisted, they could be split up, as in one will go to the BAC O'Connor Centre in Burton-on-Trent. Over-friendliness is usually determined by two persons whispering or spending excessive amounts of time together and is usually reported by their peer group. Love affairs and sexual relationships can be forged in rehab. One therapist aptly stated to all residents that the O'Connor was not a 'knocking shop' or a dating agency. It must be remembered that as well as addiction issues, residents in rehab have something else very much in common – vulnerability.

Alpha male posturing is older than the hills and is part of the species that we are or have become. At the O'Connor, though, posturing was enacted as the reason to take charge of the TV remote control (two hours a night in the week but more at the weekend). Television is a big negative in rehab. Not only does it cause friction between residents, but it can be the catalyst for the 'dumbing down' of those wanting to completely change their way of thinking. Addicts have to get out of the old ways of living their lives, which includes watching endless mindless TV. There is a strong argument that TV in rehab should be restricted to special occasions only.

One resident was so stressed by the loud TV (in both rooms at times) that when they were made captain that same resident introduced a new rule (captains can make selective decisions). To frustrate the social hierarchy and control by the few of what was watched on TV, that resident declared that the most recent resident to be admitted to the BAC would be given the remote control. If they then decided they did not want it, they could pass it on to the next newest resident, and so on and so forth. This caused hell to break loose where the atmosphere could be cut by a knife.

Some therapists at the O'Connor seemed to encourage the social structure, silently believing that the addict was progressing in taking charge of their lives by taking charge of the TV; in that by taking their responsibilities seriously in the house the residents would 'project' that responsibility in the outside world. This could be construed as a misconception. One therapist even argued that those new to rehab could not make such a tough decision as to what would be watched on TV and so should not have been given the remote control in the first place.

The resident who introduced the controversial remote control rule discharged themselves from the centre just days later. Then in 2012, that same remote control rule brought in by that same resident was made compulsory.

If you do make the decision to enter rehab you will be living with people who you do not get on with or even dislike. One has to become selfish though, because it is your recovery. Some therapists argue that rehab is a microcosm of ordinary life, in that in life you have to tolerate those you do not like. This might be so, but in real life you may have to work with people you do not get along with, but you do not have to live with them.

At times, rehab can feel like the Big Brother House, where one determines which housemate one would like to see evicted or discharged.

Inside O'Connor Part 5:
The Psychology of
Coordinated Attack

It is thought that in the UK, more than 90% of women involved in street prostitution use illegal drugs

It is believed that over twenty million people in Britain are affected in some way by drug/alcohol abuse. Families can then fracture as the addict causes havoc and the loved ones get caught up in the debris. It is not without reason that the addict pushes those that are closest to them away in the quest to be alone with their substance.

Some addicts take substances and still function. They hang on to old and tired clichés like, "I could never drink on my own". In the end that is all they want to do, as to be sociable and to converse when drinking wastes valuable time hitting the spot. What is that spot, one could ask? Is it like a hole inside the addict that they must fill? Some with addiction problems take multiple drugs or anything they can get their hands on. People rob, steal and cheat and even sell their bodies to buy crack cocaine and heroin. Prison as a deterrent is just incidental. Addicts also sabotage their futures at every opportunity. They will phone in to work intoxicated but thinking they are being clever, they will get prosecuted for drink driving or they will commit a minor misdemeanour to shed a bad light on themselves. Under the influence of drugs and alcohol people can do shameful things which reinforce their feelings of inferiority.

Ultimately they self-destruct.

At the BAC O'Connor Centre in Newcastle-under-Lyme, the residents initially learn about the triggers that kick-started their individual substance abuse. The Demon Drink is an appropriate descriptor. Addicts relay stories of battling with demons in their mind that are encouraging them to use. One addict detailed how they get 'that warm feeling' when drinking.

When starting group therapy, the group is told indirectly that not all present would necessarily be alive in two years' time. The new resident starts in small groups at first, where a therapist will focus in on any individual. In later groups residents begin to 'share', as it is known in rehab. This can be a long and compelling story that has affected the addict's emotions. The worst case scenario in these stories can be sexual abuse or even a death by someone close to the addict. The therapists take no prisoners and those not engaging with the group will be encouraged to do so or even homed in on.

Group can also see residents pointing out things to another resident, which always results in a tit-for-tat exchange. In other words, if one points out a fault in a person's character they will almost certainly return the compliment and find a fault in theirs. Whatever the tit-for-tat theories, discussion is good for the emotional wellbeing and if someone is sharing and feeling that same emotion that they felt at the time of the incident they are talking about, they can perhaps understand what was occurring at that time and move on from it. Well, that's the theory anyway.

The therapy of exposing one's rawness or deep insecurities, and the therapist pointing these frailties out, is a line of therapy that not all psychological experts concur with. Well, what's the point of doing the aforementioned in any event, in that what can be gained from making troubled souls squirm in their inferiority? Is it better to put things behind us and move on and not revisit troubled incidents in our lives that have deeply affected us? If some expert was to detail why this line of frailty therapy is beneficial to the addict one would take on board the argument; but no detailed explanation has been forthcoming and so the debate is open. One thing that can be said with certainty is that in group the residents are in a communal environment for the first time in many years, such has been the degree of isolation through substance misuse. Therefore, behavioural idiosyncrasies have to be identified.

Ganging up can occur in group and on one such occasion, one resident was castigated by most of the group members. A resident had told a story or 'shared', the essence of which was that they were criticising their parents for one thing or another. Another resident challenged the sharer that nobody is the perfect parent as in 'he who is without sin cast the first stone' (for want of better phraseology). A large section of the group criticised the outspoken resident for making this statement. Even one group member who rarely spoke out did so on this occasion. The next day a different therapist taking the group pointed out to all present the value of what the outspoken resident had said. At the end of that group, instead of crucifying the outspoken resident, those who had criticised the outspoken resident the previous day flung their arms around them and hugged the 'villain of the piece' instead. Yes, there are double standards in group and therapists can often have differing views on the positives and negatives of discussion.

It should also be remembered that some residents purposely turn their peers against them (by being outspoken, for example) so there will be no way for them to go other than out of the door to discharge. Addiction is cunning. One resident was so battered in group he had to lie down for a day or two to recover. He described emotional tension wracking his body for this duration. This same resident is still clean after five and a half years.

Split gender was also another form of group therapy, where the group was either male or female. This was to allow those who had anxieties about mentioning certain matters in the presence of another sex to fully air their concerns. It went without saying that at the BAC O'Connor Centre, the male groups were the envy of the female residents. Coincidentally, more interesting topics seemed to be discussed in an all-male environment.

Inside O'Connor Part 6: Psychosis Preferable to Tedium Vitae

Some cannabis users may have unpleasant experiences, including confusion, hallucinations, anxiety, paranoia and even psychosis depending on their mood and circumstances

It is thought by experts that cannabis is no soft drug and there are between two and five million regular users in Britain. Cannabis can induce psychosis and schizophrenia in those that use it. Delusions and feelings of being persecuted are commonplace, with heavy users reporting that they thought 'the TV was watching them', and that those featured on TV knew the cannabis user. Cannabis users were also under the delusion that they were the most important person in the world. This state of mind can perhaps be explained by a hypothesis that as one of the billions of ants on the planet we inherently feel that, by and large, we are insignificant. Cannabis can implant in the cerebral a distorted notion of self-importance, which counteracts our basic insignificance in the grand scheme of things. Therefore, instead of being aware that we are, by and large, unimportant players in world politics, with cannabis use we become the most important. Good therapy in this instance could be to convince the user that they indeed have relevance in their own personal world (or life) and those that are involved in that world with them (such as family, for example,) are very important in the scheme of things.

Distorted thinking can become even darker though, where heavy cannabis users feel that they are God or even the Devil. Although not physically addictive, cannabis can be mentally addictive; it also goes without saying that cannabis will do little harm if used infrequently. But addicts, when they like something, want more and more of that substance. The argument that cannabis only causes problems to those who are predisposed to mental health problems is negated by the fact that most of the population experiences anxiety or depression at some time in their lives. In saying the above, cannabis should be decriminalised (accompanied by wide-reaching education programmes), the reason being that the destruction caused by the legal drug alcohol, both physically and mentally, is far greater.

A standard day at the BAC in Newcastle begins at seven o'clock in the morning when one is called by the house staff. The resident then has their allotted job to perform, like hoovering the lounge. There is also a deep clean on a Sunday when ovens in the kitchen will be dragged out, for example. The resident's room also has to be deep cleaned on a Sunday and will be inspected by a member of the house staff and the resident captain, and if it is not up to scratch the resident will have to do it again. Also on Sundays, the resident's laundry is done and the captain and vice-captain make a rota to choose which resident will be allocated what job for the forthcoming week. The social pyramid can surface again at this interval, as in those that the captain likes could get the easier jobs and those that they do not could get the more unpleasant ones. Deep cleans were important, as no balanced person wants to live in squalor. It was in squalor that many addicts found themselves before deciding to enter a programme of rehabilitation.

Life can be dull at times and at the BAC O'Connor Centre, it can be just as dull. As in, when the day of therapy is over, what does one do? Many users described how their lives are/were boring before admittance and substances brought variation to their existence. Structuring one's life while at the BAC is vital if one is to remain substance-free. It is therefore paramount that outside agencies like universities/colleges and employment/voluntary groups actively engage with facilities like the O'Connor Centre. At the time of research there was very little cooperation from these agencies. Addicts struggle to get through the day and need to function in the community for a sense of wellbeing. Employment exchanges would be surprised at the 'untapped talent' that has spent years befuddled by substance misuse.

There is also a prevailing theory in rehab circles that 'there were good times' when using. One supposes this means that they had a fit of giggles with a group of friends when smoking cannabis or how everyone laughed and thought how funny it was when an individual was escorted or even barred out of a nightclub for being 'a general nuisance'. Then there was the time when one's mind 'opened up' to the hallucinogen or they danced all night and then made multiple conquests because of 'Dutch courage' or that 'loved-up' feeling. We also have those that went out to pubs and clubs just to be involved in some kind of fracas – where someone inevitably ended up in hospital or in jail. The reality is that all the so-called good times were induced by a substance.

To deal with routine in rehab is the same as dealing with routine on the outside but without substances to break up the tedium. There was no access to the Internet for the residents during their stay and one bog-standard radio was allowed in the resident's room. The workshops at the centre acknowledged structure and a sense of wellbeing as of paramount importance and offered practical actions to help instil a sense of purpose and confidence into the resident. The workshops can vary and one example was that everyone in the group gave one positive word to describe their peers and one negative word to describe them. Then all the comments were written down and given to the peer. Another workshop was that the therapist played a significant tune that the resident had selected and the resident would comment on the tune and what it meant or means to them now. This could be a poignant exercise to induce a feeling of self-worth in the addict. In contrast, the song could be chosen to enable the addict to look at their warped behavioural patterns in that particular era of their lives.

Another workshop elucidated the theoretical story regarding 'the rabbits and the elephants' which is better narrated by the therapists. The general idea is that problems are like little white rabbits. If one white rabbit was sitting next to you, you would not flinch, but if there were multiple rabbits (or problems) abounding, you would begin to become unnerved or even worried. The idea ascribes that one deals with one's problems one at a time, before they become too overpowering, not forgetting you are going to get a big elephant crossing your path at some stage (the elephant is a metaphor for an unexpected death or some significant other problem). It is thought that if you have not dealt with the rabbits the elephant could trample you to death (as in you could start using again). The residents enjoyed the theory of the rabbits and the elephant. The workshops also engender camaraderie amongst the peer group.

The 'shop run' and 'bank runs' were also part of the routine at the O'Connor Centre, where on the shop run, two residents would go to a supermarket nearby (escorted by a volunteer or a 'clean' ex-resident) to shop for listed items for the other residents. No doubt this entailed piles and piles of sugary goods and was a difficult task to both individually shop for a resident and deliver the correct change. The bank runs saw five or six residents go into Newcastle to use the banks. All the residents would stay together in a group with a member of the house staff presiding. They then, in turn, would have to visit every resident's personal bank and wait outside while the resident did their banking business. One resident described how they felt silly and childlike, all marching up to Newcastle in a little gaggle with their house staff watchman.

Throughout the 18-week period at the BAC some residents would leave and new ones would be admitted. Some would leave very close to completion of the programme. There were many reasons given by the residents why they were leaving but at the end of the day they left to use again, even if they were unaware of it at the time. One resident left after nine weeks because of friction with other residents. The resident reported that initially they had not chosen to drink when deciding to leave. Nevertheless, the resident in question asked for day care (a programme of treatment without living-in) when deciding they could not live with the other residents anymore. This was refused by the therapist. In the days leading up to the resident leaving the centre the resident then decided to use (drink alcohol in this case) once discharged. The therapist then offered the resident day care as they were just about to leave but the resident refused because by then they had already decided to use again. Therefore, this overlap, between deciding to leave and the day care option, needs greater analysis to save another addict from a similar fate.

Inside O'Connor Part 7:
This is Your Life

Addicts and therapists alike will maintain that harm by substance abuse is experienced not only by the partakers themselves, but by those around them, including families, friends, colleagues and strangers

People often cross the street at the sight of a heroin addict begging. Heroin users stand out from the crowd, not just because of their appearance or the fact they can ask for money, but by the over-familiar way they can make contact with strangers.

In the outside world, during a debate on a proposed pigeon cull, one person stated with words to the effect that it is not the pigeons that should be culled but the 'smack heads'. This is how ugly-minded and uncompassionate some people can be. These addicts are not aliens from outer space but somebody's wife, brother, husband, father, son or daughter.

As residents at the BAC O'Connor Centre near the end of their programme (week nine or ten) an important exercise is undertaken, where one has to write out one's life story. Residents were not allowed to use a computer to write their story but had to do it by hand. One then had to narrate one's life story (or read it out) to the rest of the group in the presence of one or two therapists. The therapists and some of the residents would then make observations about pivotal moments contained in the story and pose questions to the narrator after they had concluded.

Telling the story could be a difficult exercise for the resident and the psychology behind it is best explained by the ones who initiate it. One resident had a nosebleed before their life story, while another felt the same paranoia as they did whilst using cannabis.

The reasons why the life story is so important during rehab could be to 'unload burdens' or even to punctuate the mistakes in an addict's life. The strategy that fresh eyes were looking at the dysfunctional life of the addict could also be behind the exercise, as in throw new light on the triggers and life events that initially enabled the addictive lifestyle for the resident sitting.

One-upmanship can also be seen during life stories; insomuch as a small minority of addicts could revel in their gangster-like pasts; or how much of a drug they could take in comparison to someone else. Some life stories could include violence or sexual abuse, which would be difficult for the narrator to disclose. A commonality of personal traumatic events seemed to be the linking thread to bind nearly all the life stories. Conversely, there were one or two exceptions. Like the story told by one young woman who declared that a 'friend' had injected her with heroin while she was asleep.

Perhaps at this point one must also determine in one's own mind if it is good to bare the soul and discuss very personal aspects of one's life to semi-strangers. Or are some things best kept private and to oneself? The debate is open.

Writing the life story for the resident was deemed so important that they could be excused their allotted house cleaning duties when coming to the life-story part of the programme. During the 18-week programme at the O'Connor, residents would be well aware of the AA (Alcoholics Anonymous) and NA (Narcotics Anonymous) meetings on Saturday mornings before visiting time. At first the personal stories from the sitting representative from AA and NA regarding their addiction would be interesting but as one became immersed in AA/NA culture, the listeners could hear the same theme over and over again. A covert religious undercurrent seems to flow through the meetings but is never admitted. The representative addressing the group could hold a black book (which was not the Bible but looked like it). It can be argued that the O'Connor Centre overly relies on AA and NA meetings as a place for those completing the programme to go for support. There is very little help elsewhere.

Graduation is a process when the resident has completed the programme and all their relatives, the residents, staff and therapists assemble in a room for the celebration of completion. Residents can dread this event and some would discharge rather than face it. Even the new residents have to take part in this exercise, even though they barely know the resident graduating. Everyone would say a few words, as a medal of sorts is passed around from person to person. If one did not know the person one could just say 'good luck' or something like that. It seemed that graduations were always coming up at the centre and one newish resident began to resent them, not just because they were forced to talk on the spot in front of a big audience but because it was too much too soon and seemed to them to be slightly superficial. Jokes would abound with the residents before a graduation ceremony. For example, one resident in the communal lounge would pull a concerned face and mock the ceremony as in they would say something like, "Yes, I knew Joe Bloggs as a nice fellow and we will be chums for life", and in a condescending voice they would carry on to say "I remember that day when they first came in to rehab; it was a Tuesday and the weather was of a dark mood," etc. A good laugh between the residents always ensued from this mocking enactment before the graduation ceremony.

On a more serious note, graduation is viewed by the therapists as a very important component of rehabilitation and, if one does not graduate, one has failed the programme. Aftercare can only become available after graduation, whereby a resident, once having left the centre, can return for ongoing support – even if they lapse or relapse.

Finally, and as an afterthought, therapists can also give a resident extra weeks to complete at the centre if they feel the resident needs further therapy. But when all's said and done, the resident must take full responsibility for their own actions. If someone committed a violent crime against us and apologised that they could not help it because they were an addict, would we forgive them? The answer is no; addiction is an illness, not a mitigation.

Inside O'Connor Part 8: Avoid Poisonous Arenas

Some people can go out and have a good time without taking any substances at all but they are the minority. For the recovering addict it could be sensible to avoid places where narcotics are liberally dispensed, like pubs and nightclubs.

There is no one organisation that actively collects information about drug-related deaths for all of Great Britain. In other words, nobody knows exactly how many deaths there are each year linked to drug/alcohol inebriation. For example, there are no statistics on:

- people who are dependent on drugs and overdose
- suicides by overdose of people who have no previous history of using drugs
- accidental overdose
- ecstasy-related deaths where people have died from overheating through dancing non-stop in hot clubs rather than from the direct effect of the drugs
- deaths associated with cigarette smoking
- deaths from accidents where people are drunk or under the influence of drugs
- murders and manslaughters where people are drunk or under the influence of drugs
- deaths from driving while drunk or intoxicated
- deaths from Aids among injecting drug users

- deaths which had nothing to do with the presence of a drug in the body
- sexual assault or disease as a result of alcohol inebriation

What makes an addict an addict is not up for debate in these articles. Whether it's a hole in the soul, a result of a traumatic event, nature or nurture, or a mix of all the aforementioned, no one will never really know. What we do know is that addiction to substances is growing and growing in Britain today. At the O'Connor, the treatment is based on total abstinence in that substitutes for heroin, like methadone, are not allowed at all. Few rehabs offer this source of treatment, which is more than likely the reason the O'Connor has high success rates.

But is an addict still an addict if they do not use a substance full-time but drink to excess once a week? The debate opens up again but what is known is that one will have a better quality of life engaging in the latter.

Then there is the dilemma regarding explanation in the wider world context. If one was once a heavy drinker and becomes dry and is asked if they would like a drink what should they say? They should politely say, "No thank you, I don't drink." One does not buy the idea that one must explain that they are an alcoholic or similar; it's your private business, after all. Some argue that to avoid the pub and club scene is the better option because it is not always a suitable environment for those who are sober. If it is an important function and you should attend, do so for a shorter time if you find it difficult to relate to people at drink-fuelled occasions. Or if you are a driver, offer to drive instead. When an addict is celebrating they can be in danger, as a happy mood can render the addict to want and need to heighten this mood with a substance.

In the nightclub scenario or not, today people take multiple drugs. They will take crack cocaine with alcohol as an upper and then take heroin to come down. Mixing alcohol and cannabis can render one crawling on the floor for the bathroom. Other more obscure drugs are coming to the fore, like ketamine and derivatives from horse tranquillisers or weed killers. Then we have the more recent strains of black mamba, monkey dust and spice. Yes, some people feel desperately inadequate and where there is a false high there is inevitably a worse low around the corner. Most addicts are so emotionally impoverished they prefer their lives asleep, as when in slumber they are operating in a world other than this one. How do we change this?

Sustained support after rehabilitation is crucial if the addict wants to remain drug-free. Some kind of work or academic course, coupled with an interesting hobby or pursuit, can fill the vacuum and raise the chances of the addict always being substance-free. Human beings will always have addiction issues; jogging, swimming or another positive sport can be the addict's new addiction.

The legislators and educators can play their part too. Drug facts should be known so people can make an informed choice. After all, people are people and, as such, they will always take mood enhancers of some kind or another. It's no use quoting another tired old cliché like, 'everything is okay in moderation' – addicts don't do moderation.

Binge drinkers or the once or twice a week drinkers will one day realise the reason they never felt fulfilled with their lives or did not achieve what they wanted to achieve was/is down to a lack of self-confidence or lack of physical fitness brought about by binge drinking. Alcohol is so subtle in its destruction that to use it through your life, even intermittently, will still determine it. The nervous system takes a week to recover from even one sitting of consuming copious amounts, which will cause or exacerbate mental health issues like low mood, agoraphobia, panic attacks and anxiety during the days after intoxication. After a good blowout on alcohol one can take a week to fully recover and what does one do after this week? Yes, they drink again so the destructive cycle continues.

Until you decide to stop it, of course. Then you will have to rewire (or recycle) your thinking so being substance-free becomes your new habit. This will take time.

In 2017, the BAC O'Connor Centre in Newcastle-under-Lyme closed down due to funding cuts in social care. The facility in Burton-on-Trent remains open. The impact the Newcastle closure will have on the wider community will probably never be quantified.

The powers that be don't record statistics on such things.

The Celebrity Dirty Old Goat

Sexual manipulation meted out by those in privileged positions (film celebrities in this instance) has always been the case. So why all the furore regarding Weinstein and Spacey? Hasn't the capitalist ideologue always had a free run in the motion picture industry? The brutal facts are that the 'wannabes' who have designs on sharing in the film industry's out of control wealth will drop to their knees for the promise of a part. Sexual favours, used as a bargaining chip, which in turn allows them to climb the movie star ladder, has been with us since the birth of Hollywood.

Then we have the suffusing popular culture as seen nowadays: "They all wanna be a starrr," don't they? I have just drawled in my most irritating American accent. And many will do just about anything to get there. When we boil it all down; privilege, control and sex have always been inter-related. So, the more money you earn, hence the more powerful you become, henceforth, the more you are idolised by sections of the masses, hereafter, the more likely you are to control other human beings for your own selfish sexual gratification. The psychologists would say it's alpha male human nature and about spreading one's seed. I would argue the connotations are much more sinister; especially when children are involved.

In the year 1973, and as an eleven-year old, I remember a Sweet concert. For the younger readers, Sweet were a glam-rock pop group of the 1970s and were very big at the time. After the show and finding ourselves outside, some other kids called us over to the front of the Victoria Hall, where we watched in amazement as the group members walked into what must have been their dressing room. They were all so hot and exhausted after the performance, all four band members (except the lead singer) stripped naked right before our eyes. We were all gob-smacked at the time and when it was pointed out by someone inside that we were all gawping in shocked excitement through the windows outside, the curtains were hastily drawn.

This unforeseen situation was entirely innocent.

Many encounters with celebrity icons have not been so innocuous, as seen with Jimmy Savile, Max Clifford and Rolf Harris. Children are so conditioned to be so star-struck by such figures, they would not have understood exactly what was going on when being abused. 'Pushy mommies' also do little to help. This comes in the form of celeb-obsessed parents who can deploy their children to be just as conditioned to mainstream celebrity culture as they are.

The loud-mouthed bully, Clifford, still denied his crimes right up to his death in December 2017. Whereas, Savile was allowed a free run by those in authority because he was generating so much wealth for the capitalist machine. Many victims were brain-washed to believe that their idols were held in such high esteem they were untouchable; thus, they could repeatedly abuse with impunity. Nobody would believe the nobody's word over the word of a famed person – safe within the confines of the system we are governed by.

I am afraid to say that the whole ethos of portraying those on screen as some sort of super-human celestial being needs to be examined if we want to deter abuse routinely practised by those in privileged positions. The be-all and end-all of human existence also needs to be analysed, focussing on what values and false needs we are programmed to aspire to.

The media (especially the tabloid press) also perpetuate the false celebrity ideal by bombarding us with 'superstar' minutiae, as if these very fortunate individuals (some making millions for acting the dirty old goat) are so nonpareil, they are akin to demi-gods.

This medium icon old puffery misnomer also needs to be addressed.

The Wise Owl & the Sky Track

Featuring Scary Spider

"Oh what a beautiful morning," chirped Wise Owl in full song. "Oh what a beautiful day."

It had been as cold as Iceland when Wise Owl emerged from slumber. He was freshly wizened up from steeped in wisdom dream dimensions.

Today was to be Wise Owl's D for Definitive day. He had dreamt about interplanetary assembly points the night before last.

He knew his rocket science.

Wise Owl turned proudly toward his well-researched drawing plans.

He had wisely drafted a radical solution in a wizdomic sky conclusion.

Wise Owl switched on his leaking kettle.

"I had better get a move on," he chirped to himself.

His appointment was for 9.30am. What Wise Owl did not wisen in his wisdom was that he was about to be brought down to earth with a thundering…

CRASH…

Wise Owl opened the curtains and shrieked, aghast; it wasn't about to be a beautiful morning and it wasn't about to be a beautiful day.

Scary Spider was also awakened. Yes, he wasn't quite pleased with being disturbed from hibernation, and found it hard to focus. Scary knew, though, that something very fiendish was about to occur.

Outside, the window cracked with cold and little Scary Spider scuttled from his web in the windowsill corner. He was the first to see there had been a major transport trauma.

Earlier, noise twiggings had occurred in the dark pitch-black night before, whence Scary Spider's little hairs on his back legs had stood on edge. Shell-shocked from the experience, Scary Spider recoiled in horror at the terrifying human madwoman, screaming piercingly in recognition of him.

Scary Spider would never again mistakenly cross the wrong path.

He had made it by a whisker and had lost a little spindly leg in the process.

Scary Spider had relived the cracking foot-crushing nightmare of Scuttly Spider's demise.

Simmering thick black smoke billowed and spilled upwards in a slow circular motion. Scary Spider scarily doomed prophetically as the cold black night faded into the even colder black day. The laws of the jungle legislated that there had been drunken wild beasts on the loose the night before last; of a human kind.

Der der der der der der; the fire engine screeched in the distance eerily afar. It would be a record call out this time around for Proud Lion.

Wise Owl and Scary Spider both wised up and decided to absorb the drama from the safety of the window once they saw the lightning flash. It was safer that way.

After all, a rather large crowd was beginning to muster. Wise Owl had always wizened that it was somewhat strange and unwise to peer and prod at other souls' misfortunes.

Wise Owl had recalled witnessing the death of his dear friend and wished he hadn't. The Tasmanian Devil had feverishly scrapped around for pieces of last will and testimony in the hospital death chamber. Wise Owl was most shocked, imagining in recall, those gathered around the bed of the dying soul and those ghouling, leaning over, to stare into death without shame. The Bone-Picking Buzzard had overlooked proceedings, pencil and notebook in hand, totting up funeral costs. A licking one's lips noise sounded, heard on this occasion, parched but dry.

Wise Owl wised by the wreckage that things were not going according to plan. The driver of the metal contraption sat by the roadside; he was of road rage deposition.

The arrogant-appearing pig-headed Road Rage Hog had been doing ninety miles an hour. He had a piggish, red, nasty uncaring aggressive mein, enacting vulgar hand gestures at passing motorists.

Road Hog held head in his arms, the only consolation coming from Busy Body Bee, who would get involved in any lack-lustre drama to excite her sad life. But this cataclysmic episode was the biggest drama ever for Busy Body Bee. And she would savour and relish every moment buzzing around over the pot of misery.

Road Hog was wishing he had never been born, on looking through his hands at the decapitated head (from the car accident) rolling down the gutter and landing right before his lap. It was as though it had occurred in another surreality.

"In a parallel world there was a resolution. The Armed with Education Tiger was primed for civil malfunction."

The overturned car wreckage and smouldering smoke had mustered other Busy Body Bees buzzing for a round of curtain twitching. There was fearful dread in the air.

Proud Lion entered the fray for stamina/staying powered by agility prowess. He was one fit wild cat. The strong muscular fire officer protruded both head and defined arm out of the fire engine window, lion tails flailing out the back. His mane blew with the speed velocity of the vehicular air pressure.

Proud Lion emitted a ferocious roar that shook the whole established foundation. Grey dust cleared to slowly focus on the accident picture. An illustration of the new Sky Track, ever so slightly materialising in Wise Owl's mind's eye, now came into view.

There was a safe alternative.

Wearing an armband and smirking cunningly, sneaky-faced, Fly Fox presses the crush button: he chuckled at the slyness of the booby-trapped motor car crusher interring the metal underground. Emblazoned on the side of the crusher was the company name and slogan: 'ClearingRoadDeaths: Saving Lives with road reforestation'.

Alongside and slightly out of perspective, there could be seen a strange vehicle Sky Track construction, big dipper-like, that crossed overground. Metal motor contraptions whizzed in navigation over it at some speed.

Was that a fun ghost train variation of the Sky Track over yonder?

The corpses involved in the accident were taken away. So Wise Owl quickly donned his woolly wise hat and coat and decided to head for the hospital mortuary, where he knew they would be chilled in storage. He was on to something. He could sense it in the air. He would see the fallout for himself.

"Aghh," shrieked Wise Owl with a shiver, as he cast his frightened wise eyes on a body in the heavy refrigerator door.

Wise Owl stood at the hospital morgue drawer pull, viewing the refrigerated inhumane Human Being character, identity tag on ankle. There was a medical-looking sign, saying, 'Cold meat chilling.'

Shock tactics.

"There's one a day," echoed the heavy-breathed doctor Weird Wolf in slow hushed tones, silhouetted in the candlelight of the dimly-lit laboratory.

"The casualty rate's twinned with Birmingham, Alabama, you know," he drawled in his West Bronx accent.

"'Death by Cold Steal' car thief, this one." The Weird Wolf laughed weirdly and wolfishly; a demonic chortle almost.

Peculiar Pelican, donned his befitting mortuary attendant's coat, pulled open the cold slab drawer with a banging swooshing motion. *Was that a cigarette Peculiar Pelican was smoking, or was he testing his own peculiar temperature?* Wise Owl pondered.

Feathers descended slowly and eerily out of another steel tray.

"This one was brought in just yesterday," Peculiar Pelican very matter of factly peculiarised with Weird Wolf. In condensed breath the scientific and climatic observational discursive analytics were very interesting... delineating over biological grey matters and black lung, shall we just say.

"Isn't peculiar a peculiar word?" Peculiar Pelican was overheard to say from a distance.

It had been the usual scenario concerning road death occurrence. It was readily accepted like the common cold. Okay as long as it does not affect you personally.

Could it ever change? Wise Owl puzzled, while purchasing his morning bannocks from the bakers the very next day. He tossed a few morsels to the Scavenging Pigeon as he strolled out of the shop. The setting quickly switched to a previous and it was another dull and monotonous day, predictable in its predictability. Monday morn, Wise Owl's foot was incarcerated with a ball and chain. The owl held life instructions in hand. It read:

'This is what your betters determine; you must comply.'

There was bureaucratic junk mail piled up on the owly-faced doormat. The verdict was that the daring Sky Track was all in Wise Owl's wise and idealist mind.

Fantastical futures were just a mere consciousness away. But this was the grim reality; humanimal suffering for blood money is the name of the game today.

Pollution, like tragic roundabouts, loses lives, maniacs driving around in circles and Death… abounds every corner; it bites hard, sinks deep and takes your last breath.

Wise Owl in his wisdom had no choice but to plummet disastrously downbeat. The environment was polluting his brain, and he needed to lie down and collect his thoughts. The world was an unsafe and austere place, he quickly reasoned, and no place for the wise and the more civilised of the species.

The same occurrence recurred later that morning during Wise Owl's interview with officialdom; negative know-alls were an understatement. With drawings in hand, Wise Owl had wisely observed the same re-enactment countless times before. It had seemed predictably odious how Big Negative Nellie the Elephant always seemed to know best. *Nellie-know-all*, thought Wise Owl, tucked up in his safe hole for the winter, reflecting on another empty day.

Wise Owl decidedly attempted to cook dinner and before long saucepans were bubbling harmoniously and slowly in his little, but wise, back kitchen. It was skate and kiddly pie, his favourite, tonight. Wise Owl served his meal and put out Scary Spider's minute portion and tucked tentatively in, with slow stressed motions. Then, right out of the blue, a rather banal wise thought occurred him.

"Nothing ever changes and nothing ever ends," he whispered aloud in his very wise head.

"It's just the same every day."

Wise Owl wisely pushed the whys and wherefores back to the recesses of his wise evolving mind. He would leave that conundrum to the so-called experts to decipher.

As Wise Owl began to tuck with more vigour into his skate and kiddly pie, a nauseating comparison concluded.

He had witnessed Hare Rabbit's cousin Harriet's demise. The roadside left her squashed giblets for months after. It had been a truly devastating experience for the O'Hare family.

Would we all have to carry on dying on the roads indefinitely? Wise Owl wisely pondered in a wise but confused conclusion.

Wise Owl suddenly did not feel very hungry. Instead, he switched on his electric blanket. It had been one dire day. He started to wisely circumnavigate his little map of Jupiter imprinted on his square, not round, bulbous lamp.

He began reading in bed, earth-shattered and yawning by the light of his Jupiter lamp, warmth emanating from the electric blanket, heating up his little wise bed. Wise Owl stared at the night sky in disbelief (through the roof window telescope).

Scary Spider simultaneously snuggled up under his silken webbed eiderdown. Nightcap atop, he looked quite hard done by. The good news was that his missing leg was already starting to grow back. He sighed in painful relief.

Scary Spider's voice broke.

"Is there anything you don't know, Wise Owl?"

"Yes," retorted Wise Owl, in his wisest voice.

"I don't know what devastation the greedy chaotic humans are going to bring tomorrow. But I do know one thing; with Polly Ution in the ascendancy, nothing will change for the better."

With this, Scary Spider yawned and snuggled down to go to sleep. He was snoring before long.

The world had crumbled the day the Sky Track proposal fell through.

Scuttly Spider and the inhumane Human Being had perished unnecessarily, too.

Lowry Didn't Care Much Anyway

An interesting day out can be experienced by a visit to The Lowry on Salford Quays, Greater Manchester. Free to go in, the number 50 bus from Albert Square, Central Manchester (outside the Slug and Lettuce) will take you straight to the gallery.

In the actual Lowry building, theatre shows are also staged and in the same complex there can be found a tourist information desk, together with the customary refreshments facility.

Always remembering that 1978 hit, *Matchstalk Men and Matchstalk Cats and Dogs* by Brian and Michael, who this Lowry character actually was has always drawn me.

Born in Stretford, the obscure and complex Laurence Stephen Lowry (1887–1976) was as enigmatic as some of his paintings, the more familiar being the masses of matchstick men against the backdrop of urban and industrial poverty-stricken northern life, set in the early to mid-20th century.

Lowry's personal life (according to the twenty-minute film at The Lowry) is far more compelling. His domineering mother would affect the psychological wellbeing of her to-be-famous son with her constant belittling tongue.

Described as asexual by his student friends, Lowry didn't care much for intimacy and was a solitary and withdrawn figure who made few lasting relationships. It is well documented that he concentrated instead on caring for his bedridden mother for eight years of his life until her death in 1939.

More alarmingly, the twenty-minute screening at The Lowry, references a Securicor van visiting Lowry's home after his demise to take away the famous paintings. However, this part of the film can be confusing as it was not understood what the significance was.

Mysteries aside, The Lowry is a great place to visit and houses some of the artist's paintings and drawings that have never before been seen in the public domain. My personal favourites are: *Going to the Match* (1928) and *Street Scene* (1935).

The Cold War

Thirty years ago, if someone had posed the theory that you should not go to hospital because you might catch a virus that could kill you, they would have been laughed out of court. The laughs would have been even haughtier if one dared to suggest that some people are afraid that super bugs like C. diff and MRSA have been orchestrated to 'finish off' those who are a strain on the health service, like the old folk. Then we had Stafford Hospital.

And for the decriers or those in denial out there, yes, there can be experienced pockets of professionalism within our hospitals, but generally they are a mess.

At ground level, the concept of feeling a drain on our NHS is never far away from the fore of many older people's conscious. Conspiracy theories or not, what I can tell you is that the infectious diseases abounding in the health service today are man-made, in that resources to guard against these infections can prevent them from occurring; prevention is better than the cure. No funding for hygiene manpower spells disaster. So yes, nobody can deny that the current epidemics sweeping the health service are man-made. In the Netherlands, where they spend a little more on hygiene, bugs are isolated immediately. This is probably because sections of the Dutch government still have a social conscience and a responsibility to protect the wider public.

The latest 'plague' to hit the British Isles is the norovirus, where one is advised to stay at home, metaphorically daub a red cross on one's door and wait for it to pass.

Another common virus not talked about too often, and the one everybody is catching, isn't necessarily known as being dangerous, but that's just what it is. The common cold will breach the hardiest immune system and you will receive no succour. A cough or a sneeze by another passenger on the bus sends others running for cover, such is the guile of this clever microorganism. Sore throat, runny nose, and body ache – you name it, you'll get it. This bug has such a devious mind of its own, when you think you have shaken it off, it cleverly returns to put you through the same agony all over again. I don't know about what anybody else thinks but these are strange times, in which, for older people, the common cold can weaken the immune system where it can evolve into flu, or even pneumonia, which inevitably brings about a death sentence for those infected.

Those worldwide who die directly as a result of the common cold cannot be quantified.

I tried my own remedy to deter the dreaded cold lurgy after the flu jab failed to prevent a couple of nasty cold outbreaks during the winter months of 2016. In 2017, from late September until mid-May, I drank the juice of a fresh lemon every day and did not suffer from a cold.

I wonder if it was just coincidental.

Cool Christmas

To use a Potteries' idiom, I am not 'nesh', but I do like to keep warm indoors. Notwithstanding, I recently discovered that to keep my home cosy comes at great cost.

In paying £36 per week for electricity and with winter now all-pervading, I naturally enquired of my supplier why the electric bill was so high.

By my own admission, I could leave the immersion heater on for longer than one was supposed to, the electric blanket could be switched on indefinitely (yes when you think life is tough it can feel a lot tougher if you're getting into a cold bed at night). In addition, the heater in the bathroom would have to be on before yours truly would use the shower and I always made sure it was nice and snug in the living room while using my computer.

I was also misinformed that halogen heaters are inexpensive to run and would switch mine on willy-nilly.

Cold is a pain, I would always argue, not realising that I was about to literally experience just how unpleasant it can be.

After telephoning the electricity company and relaying the same security information three times, coupled with the customary holding (that and reading those nasty little kilowatts on your meter can render one grey overnight), I did manage to speak to a staff member at the Energywise Team. This unit is designed to divulge information with regard to how much individual electric appliances cost to run.

When I was informed that the heaters were costing a fortune, and it costs 61p an hour for the immersion to heat up water in the day time and 19p early morning, a serious chill ran down my spine.

I had been heating the water up at peak rate like there was no tomorrow.

Yes, it was therefore concluded that it would be all change at Kev's Bat Cave. I set my immersion heater to the lower heating times (those who do not engage in home cooking can boil a kettle for the dishes) my electric blanket goes on one hour before bedtime and the halogen heater is now defunct.

There is nothing like losing money to action that catalyst for change, is there?

In saying that, I was about to discover that to save on energy can be detrimental to your sense of wellbeing.

It can be a health hazard not being able to open windows for fresh oxygen to circulate; afraid it will render the room on a parallel with the Arctic Circle. This means that one will constantly be breathing in carbon dioxide. Although you can turn down the heating and wrap a warm duvet around you in the living room, you still have to move around from one chilly chamber to another.

Not being able to turn the heating on in the bathroom before a shower is also extremely uncomfortable and affects morale (no, I refuse to give that 'luxury' up).

In essence, who knows how many out there are living in freezing homes and as a result contracting infections and flu viruses because of it. Statistically speaking, fuel poverty kills 3,000 people in Britain every year.

There is talk of bringing energy companies back into public ownership and the sooner the better as far as I am concerned. It's not so long ago that the constant hikes in billing sent many of us spiralling towards the edge.

What sort of society are we living in when those working full-time have to resort to using a duvet to keep warm on an evening?

Furthermore, what are the elderly, the vulnerable and those on low incomes going through?

Talking of which, if you are in receipt of benefits you can apply for the £140 government 'Warm Home Discount'. It comes as a one-off payment every year but you had best apply to your supplier around March.

Skip a few more months to September and more misery can be declared. Yes, it's approaching Christmas time. What's even worse, some would say it's as Dickensian as it's always been (without the top hats). At this time of year many face unburdened debt attempting to keep up with the predominant materialist culture by sporting the same old standardised commodities but larger.

Just like the predictable seasonal bug, at Xmas time the health service resembles the old work house and we have the threat on our already stretched to breaking point emergency services who now have to accommodate the quagmire of alcohol-induced domestic battles sometimes occurring when something is drunkenly blurted out which had festered the whole year. It's called emotional overspill. Not to leave out our social services, of course, who are in fact, more of a metaphor for the old pauper's poor box where they want you to put in not take out.

Like the predictability of the accompanying tinsel to the festive tree, this time of year only offers more road traffic deaths, due to the pathetic ritualistic office parties when for some, it's the only time they would become inebriated. Then there's the increase in nervous breakdowns and suicide rates, when the penny finally drops for some that in reality, they have got nothing at all.

We may not be able to predict the White Christmas scenario, but for some, a Black Christmas is a real seasonal inevitability.

Then we have the modern-day street urchins come heroin addicts, with the latest being, when you don't give, "God Bless", just in case it pulls at your heart strings as you are walking away, so you turn around to donate to their drug cause. In fact, the last thing they want from you is a cup of tea or something to eat. Consequently, it would not offend to offer to buy them a sandwich, or better still, offer to refer them to an agency/clinic for treatment (if there are any left open). Today, in 2018, homelessness appears to be rising; the evidence is visible on the streets.

It's the same old Christmas message for the New Year, isn't it? Get into debt, further line the already deep pockets of the few and drink to excess the drug called alcohol which will, in turn, help us concentrate on the negative. After all, dysfunctional societies are easier to control that way. It appears that many don't quietly sup wine and absorb the cultural festivities during this time of year. They can become more uncouth than ever.

We also have the single parents who have to feed and clothe their offspring during this time of year. Then there are the seniors in our society as described above; who will be lucky to turn on their heating as the winter chill creeps into their bones. Imagine the Scrooge scenario, frightened, mittened fingers slowly scratching at the threatening envelope reminder, in fear of another salivating wolf at the door. Nice time Christmas is, isn't it? The bright side being; we can always watch the excellent *Scrooge* (1951) starring Alistair Sim as the old miser; with a view to the fact that things could be worse.

A false crimson glow akin to the slow flush of the mulled wine can encompass staff at stores around this time of year. All encouraged, of course, via Christmas songs blaring out of department store loudspeakers. Suddenly, staff are ultra-personable; after all it's the season of goodwill, not a marketing direction from management to feed the ego so we will part with more seasonal shillings. Talking of false jollification and edacious festivities, the religious significance of Xmas is never even up for debate for the majority. Folk just immerse themselves inside a tinselled, colourful space of make believe, insulated against the cold light of day. And who can blame them? Life can be harsh.

One can remember not so long ago when pubs and clubs on Christmas Eve and New Year's Eve were jam-packed. In those days one had to have tickets and paid the earth to get into a venue. There were partygoers en masse and one would not want to miss it for the world. The 'bouncers' would hold a bucket at the venue door and you were expected to drop in a pound or two for the privilege of entrance. Oh, how times have changed. Now the proprietors of such establishments would need to pay you to enter their clubs, such has been the demise of pub and club culture over the seasonal period.

Remembering Christmas as a child, not being able to sleep on Christmas Eve because of over-excitement and then waking up on that special day to unwrap one's presents was a feeling unmatched in a lifetime. Christmas is for children; they should enjoy it while they can.

And if the going gets tough this Christmas, never mind, you can always console yourself with a seasonal favourite:

Christmas is coming
The goose is getting fat (we used to say: 'and the Pigs are getting fat')
Please put a penny in the old man's hat
If you haven't got a penny, an ha'penny will do
If you haven't got a ha'penny
God bless you.

Passing the Bus

I don't live cocooned from the realities of life. I do not shield myself from the harshness of the area I live in by the luxury of financial detachment either.

I have visited hospitals, care homes, and addiction centres and I engage with energy companies, Internet providers, councils, courts, medical experts and ombudsmen. Yes, I know what's going on out there. How these companies/institutions managed the one of taking monies out of our accounts (direct debit) heaven knows. Then, if a wrong amount is taken, or they have not provided a service you have paid for, it can be a distressing battle to get your own money back. Yours truly always asks for a goodwill gesture for the anxiety caused. The more professional companies/ institutions always oblige, especially when I declare that they have not given me anything; all I have achieved is getting my own money back which is a failure demand in causing me unnecessary and undue anxiety through no fault of my own.

Failure demands aside, I have never before felt so ashamed and so fired up to complain as I was some years back when using public transport. The incident in question was regarding the free bus pass for the elderly.

I was travelling on a bus when it stopped and an elderly lady got on. As she sat down, the bus driver called to her that it was not yet 9.30am, so she must pay a fare or leave the bus.

He had allowed her on by mistake.

Another passenger exclaimed in disgust that we were talking thirteen minutes because by my watch the time was 9.17am precisely.

The woman sheepishly alighted the bus in the pouring rain and began to walk the rest of the way into town.

Disgusted is not quite the right word; try adding ashamed and sickened to live under a council that could inflict that insult on anyone, let alone an elderly person. Due to age, many can forget the half-nine rule.

For council officials to penny-pinch like this from older people in bringing in a prerequisite that they cannot use their free bus passes until after 9.30 defies all human grace.

Especially in light of the fact older people get up much earlier and so can be made housebound until 9.30am because of it. When I have brought this to the notice of council leaders, reminding them of the 9.30 ruling, they are not even shamed. I have also asked why the ruling has not been abolished. A superficial list response ensued, with regard to all the councils' 'achievements' so far. Abolishing the 9.30 rule was not one of those achievements.

As of October 2018, the ruling is still in place.

On a different note, but in the same vein it can be argued that those who use public transport gain that extra insight into real life. What has also been witnessed on more than one occasion on local buses is that elderly people are mislaying their bus passes due to age. Ruthless drivers on orders from their bosses then make the elderly person pay.

This is in light of the fact that one elderly person said in mitigation to the driver after mislaying her pass, "Don't I look sixty or seventy?" while another said, "The bus driver even knows me." When witnessing such repugnance, I asked the driver why he is taking money from those who he knows have passes and are obviously pensioners. I asked him if he was a jobsworth and told him it's bad what he is doing, to which he did not respond.

That same elderly lady who had mislaid her bus pass also stated to others on the bus that she does not like to go out because she feels so hateful towards the system. She went on to say that she has worked all her life for her bus pass, to then be charged for mislaying it. She subsequently found her pass minutes later while still on the bus, but it was too late according to the bus driver, she was told to visit the office for a refund (more stress). I heard it all. The feeling of resentment showed by this woman is endemic up and down the country, felt by the age group that vote. Do we want to live in a society like this? Deep down, even those who do well out of this failing system know something is very, very wrong.

Around the Wrekin to Get a Hearing

Due to government cuts, to file a claim oneself as a Litigant Acting in Person (LIP) at County Court has become an unmitigated nightmare where many are struggling for some sort of semblance of justice.

HM Courts and Tribunals Services nationally, have cut counter staff which has caused widespread pandemonium, particularly in the family courts.

These cuts have seen a shift where now small claims have to be filed in Salford and heard in Northampton if you are resident in Stoke-on-Trent.

Confusing, isn't it?

It is also worth remembering that if your claim (including fee remission) is not in order or in date it will be returned.

One claimant applying to the Small Claims Court had their application sent back four times because court staff did not fully understand the substituted service and serving out of jurisdiction rules.

To make matters worse, we then have that ambiguous and technically sterile language used by some judges on the court orders which is another setback for the layman acting in person. However, those filing applications at Stoke-on-Trent County Court are fortunate in a sense. The Community Legal Companion (Clock) has been set up in the foyer of the Bethesda Street building most mornings to assist those embroiled in the bureaucratic quagmire surrounding legal applications. Law students from Keele University man the front desk to assist those struggling to understand and file court applications (as of October, 2018).

It should be said that the team only offer procedural and not legal advice; and sometimes there is a fine line between legal and procedural. 'Clock' can arrange paperwork for those attending hearings, take notes at court sittings and also help with complex application forms.

What's more, their remit includes assessing if one is entitled to legal aid, advising on divorce and family matters and assisting with debt and administration applications.

Dispelling those Moscow Myths

Visiting other places around the world can expand cultural awareness. Costing as little as £100 for a return flight from Manchester or London to Moscow; visiting the Russian capital was too good an opportunity to miss. Before you rush to book though, you should be made aware that the compulsory visa to enter Russia costs over £100, the 'Invitation' (which is a prerequisite for admission to Russia) costs about £14 (2013) and the hotels can be very expensive too. As of 2018, visa regulations have become even more complex, due to Russia–UK relations.

Having learnt all about the Russian Revolution (1917) and collectivisation at high school, I was a little disappointed when in the 1980s, Russia became, well, exactly like the rest of the Western world. It was also documented that in the clash of ideologies between East and West the West had become the victor. Whatever the politico-historical past, history is infinite and the last hundred years are nothing really in the great historical scheme of things. That was history; now let's look at propaganda.

We all have preconceived ideas of a place before we have visited, which has no doubt been forged by external influences such as the media. One such myth is the idea that Russian women are all a little on the rough side – peroxide blondes, desperate for that elusive rich Westerner. This is one of the bigger mistruths, as Russian women possess a unique class of their own and can compete in the beauty stakes the world over.

There is of course another fallacy; that Moscow is just a cold, dark, austere place. On the contrary, Moscow has beautiful summers with temperatures as high as 30 degrees.

Then we have 'Ten Ton Kemp' selling us the Moscow gangster stories.

In reality, Moscow is pretty safe and the gangsters' paradise portrayed by Ross Kemp seems to be kept within its own realms and is detached from the mainstream of Russian society.

Another myth is that Muscovites are rude and miserable. The vast majority I met were accommodating, polite and helpful. When asking for directions and navigating the warren of underground passages signposted in the Russian alphabet (the English equivalent for place names is not displayed on the metro) many went out of their way to help and some even personally showed me which way to go.

Perhaps to ask younger people for directions, as they are more likely to have a better command of the English language, is the best way forward. It must be said, though, that you might get the odd older Russian who might reply to a polite request with, "Nooo Engleees". If this is the case, use all powers of restraint and composure in not doing anything you might later regret. For example, when putting up one finger to indicate how many metro tickets you would like, don't stick up two instead.

Note: not for the faint-hearted – only the hardiest of travellers should negotiate the Moscow underground challenge.

On the down side, yes, there does seem to be an abundance of grim high-rise flats in Moscow in proportion to other cities of the world. In stating the obvious, one does not believe that the likes of Nokia, Pepsi, Sharp, McDonald's and other Western conglomerates now resident in Russia will solve the massive housing conundrum with a 100-year plan any day soon. Politics aside, the object of the exercise for me personally was the visit to Red Square and Lenin's Mausoleum, where the embalmed Soviet founder (1870–1924) is lying in state – and it did not disappoint.

The queues can seem daunting at first, but on average it will take about 20–30 minutes to enter the tomb. There is, of course, the option to pretend you own the place. As in, march (or even do the military goosestep) to the front of the queue, hoping not to cause a diplomatic incident with the hordes of tourists by doing so.

One should also be aware that parts or all of Red Square and the Kremlin can be closed off at any interval without warning.

On entering the crypt, it is a little spooky where the silhouette of the uniformed guard appears to merge into the darkened entrance. A stern-looking representative with the Russian flag used as an armband then awaits you at the bottom of the steps.

Yes, it was so exciting, I entered Lenin's Mausoleum twice and could not help but wonder what it must have been like to enter the tomb when the Soviet flag was used as the armband. Now I bet that was thrilling.

Extinction a Real Possibility for the Labour Party in 2015

As Jeremy Corbyn, the alternative to austerity candidate, nudged ahead in the opinion polls for the election of the new Labour Party leader in July 2015, some odd statements came to the fore. We had Phoney Tony (Blair) who had more than likely just flown in from Sir Cliff's in Barbados to inform us that Labour cannot be elected with a 'left' agenda. On cue, titters from a select audience were heard after he cracked some joke regarding heart transplants and the fact that the Tories would be happy with a left-wing Labour Party leader – 179 British military personnel fatalities together with 500,000 Iraqi deaths is no laughing matter. Neither is the thousands of British Military personnel suffering from PTSD (post-traumatic stress disorder) as a direct result of this bogus war.

Then we had our own Little Lord Fauntleroy in Tristram Hunt (no I am not going to stoop so low as to name-call him an 'Educated Twit'). A staunch supporter of the Conservative Party plot to remove Libyan leader Colonel Gadaffi in 2011; just look at the mess Libya is in now. Apparently Mr Hunt also advocated that victory for Jeremy Corbyn would result in Labour being reduced to a pressure group.

The truth of the matter is that if the Labour Party members had appointed Mr Hunt's favourite and also in the race for leader, Liz Kendall (who is so pink on the political colour spectrum she displays a hint of Tory blue) or any of the other contenders, the Labour Party would have become extinct in England just like it had become defunct in Scotland. Yvette Cooper and Andy Burnham hardly inspired hope, difference, novelty factor or dynamism either, bearing in mind all of them did not vote against the Tory welfare cuts.

And what about the Labour MPs in North Staffordshire who also did not vote against those same Tory welfare reforms which attack the vulnerable. Mr Paul Farrelly (MP for Newcastle-under-Lyme) was one of the 184 Labour MPs who did not vote against the Tory Welfare Bill which included abolishing legally binding child poverty targets, cuts to child tax credits, reductions in ESA and phasing out housing benefit for youngsters. All sitting Stoke-on-Trent MPs, including that same mould of Ruth Smeeth, Rob Flello and Tristram Hunt, together with Paul Farrelly abstained on the vote. It appears that they have learnt nothing since Labour's brutal annihilation at the 2015 general election. At that election, all the Stoke-on-Trent seats were held with a reduced majority (with only a 51.5 % turnout in Hunt's Stoke Central constituency) while Labour's Farrelly scraped past the post in Newcastle by a whisker.

Now sit down all you so-called political know-alls and to use a local expression 'shut your stupid mouths' for a minute while I try to explain why Labour lost the 2015 general election in such a decisive fashion. Firstly, and perhaps most importantly, was the poor decision to select the uncharismatic Ed Miliband as Labour Party leader. He was not prime minister material. The Labour Party's policies were also lacking any ideological basis and what they did campaign on had, by and large, already been covered by the Tories.

Secondly, was electorate fear that the Scottish Nationalists would dictate policy in England if Labour formed a government by making an alliance with that same SNP. This was exploited mercilessly by the Conservatives.

Thirdly, Labour's lax immigration stance and pro-European Union policies lost them many votes.

Finally, little came from Labour regarding how they would inspire small-and medium-sized business with tax incentives. The party could have also expanded on how they would marry big business/wealth creation with social responsibility, as in, account for the human drive to compete and better oneself, but simultaneously factor in the importance of retaining a social conscience.

Why Labour lost the election had nothing to do with economic policy or that other nonsense regarding some debt they presided over in their last term. The masses of bread and butter Labour voters don't even know what the economy is and some would argue they don't want to know. When in that polling booth ordinary people (the majority of the population) vote on gut instinct, tradition and who they think will better their lives.

There will always be those who flit from Tory to Labour and vice versa because their corresponding political mindset is one of the same. In saying that, the masses have yet to influence the final outcome, taking into consideration that 34% of those registered did not bother to vote for any of the parties in the last general election (for those not registered the figures are more obscure).

In fact, voter turnout has steadily declined over the post-war years from 83.9% in 1950 to 59.4% in 2001. The turnout at the general election of 2015 was 66.1%.

The SNP managed to persuade those who do not usually vote to do so in the Scottish referendum on independence. The same can be done in England with a concerted and coordinated effort by those who strive for change.

If Jeremy Corbyn had not become the Labour leader there would have remained a huge vacuum for a political alternative to austerity (note I did not fall into the media trap of calling socially responsible policies anti-austerity policies). Political alternatives to austerity are gathering momentum the world over as more and more of the population are beginning to realise that austerity really means shifting even more capital from the have-nots to those who already have.

What's more, there is a desire for something new in the broader political sphere.

In conclusion, the best advice one can offer the Labour Party is to accept that Scotland has gone, in twenty years' time Wales will probably go too, so party activists need to concentrate on building a new party up from grass roots here in England – now. If they do not, a new English Party will eventually supersede it, sooner rather than later.

As for our local 'Gang of Four' (Tristram, Ruth, Rob and Paul) have they ever thought of re-forming the SDP?

Unravelling Local History
on Ford Green

Having lived in Bradeley (Stoke-on-Trent) in the early 1980s, I was very familiar with Smallthorne Bank (Ford Green Road). Instead of walking up the steep Stratheden Road and on to Bankhall Road en route to Smallthorne roundabout, it was easier to walk down Hayes Street and along Chell Heath Road. One could then catch the brown and cream Turner's double decker at the bottom of Smallthorne Bank to Hanley/Brown Edge or the Newcastle/ Ball Green double-decker to Burslem. You could also walk into Burslem from Bradeley by carrying on up Stratheden Road on to Bluestone Avenue then you would hit High Lane/Hamil Road.

Across from the bus stop at the bottom of Smallthorne Bank there also used to be a paper shop where I would buy my midget gems and the late edition of my old local paper broadsheet for the national football results (and attendances) on a Saturday evening.

It can also be recalled that my first and only car (the red bomber), which was a second-hand Mini bought for £80, has associations with Ford Green Road. I would be seen bombing around Bankhall Road in the Bradeley/ Smallthorne roundabout vicinity. Talking of which, some things never change, the roundabout was notorious to negotiate then and still holds that same notoriety today.

I never did visit Ford Green Hall while resident in Bradeley or even when my parents lived in Smallthorne (which was once known as a chapelry in Norton-in-the-Moors parish and constituted in 1859). This was in light of the fact that I was fascinated with the film *Witchfinder*

General (1968) starring Vincent Price, which was themed in a like period to the Hall.

Only costing £6.50 for a family ticket, Ford Green Hall was built as a farmhouse in 1624 and is well worth a visit. The most interesting and amusing aspects of the house are the kitchen (added in 1734) and the upstairs bedchamber ensuite with a very unusual chamber pot. Once upon a time, the unobtrusive but proud residents who wanted to spend a penny in the bedroom camouflaged the convenience to appear as though it was a set of drawers.

The biggest mystery of the Smallthorne experience relates to an old photograph of a linear row of houses on Smallthorne Bank I had acquired. I would guess that the photograph was taken at the turn of the 20th century so I decided to engage in some detective work myself and match the old row of houses with today's equivalent.

On first glance at the old photo it could not be deduced whether the photograph was taken at the top, the middle, or the bottom of Ford Green Road.

Consequently, before visiting Ford Green Hall, which is situated at the bottom of Ford Green Road, I took some up-to-date snaps at the top of the bank thinking I had located the exact row of houses.

After the tour of the Hall, and waiting for the bus in exactly the place I used to catch the old Sammy Turners, the heavens opened up and as I watched the driving rain teeming down, I noted where the real location of the row of houses on the old photograph were sited.

But what threw me out was the fact that on closer inspection of the original old photograph the main building on the row of houses was the Swan Inn public house. But where was the pub now? It was at that crossing that I became determined to crack the case and eventually located a story online dated November 2013 which featured local furore regarding the Swan Inn pub being boarded up.

So what had happened to the Swan Inn?

I then scrutinised the street sign seen on the old photograph and matched it up with Regina Street (which is a right-hand turning going down towards the bottom of Smallthorne Bank). On my return to Smallthorne it was noticed that the main Swan Inn building situated at the forefront of the row of houses now appeared to be an ordinary corner house but with the same black door. As such, it had to be deduced at which vantage point

I should take the new photograph to correspond with the row of houses in the old photograph.

Perspectives aside, the roof on both the old and new main building (the former Swan Inn) gave the game away – I had solved the mystery.

The moral to the story is that when deciding to visit our local attractions other interesting events/incidents/experiences can present which is the essence of what rediscovering local history is all about.

History is not just about immortalising establishment-ascribed heroic bourgeoisie figureheads; it is about ordinary local people like you and me. What's more, as we move forward in life, to understand our past is commensurate to understanding our present and our future in an increasingly complex world.

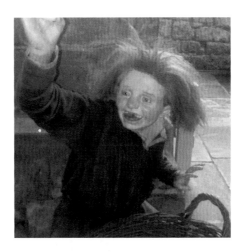

Egg on the Face of First Buses
(Page 9)

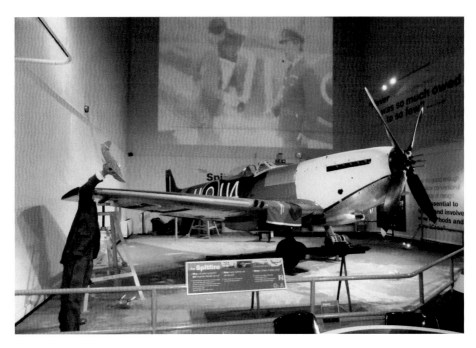

The Battle for Britain
(Page 17)

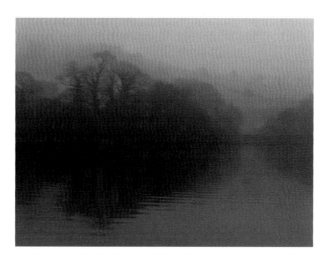

The Blurring of the Lines
(Page 20)

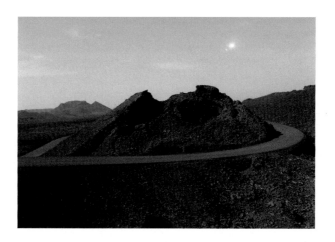

Trick Photography in Lunarote
(Page 25)

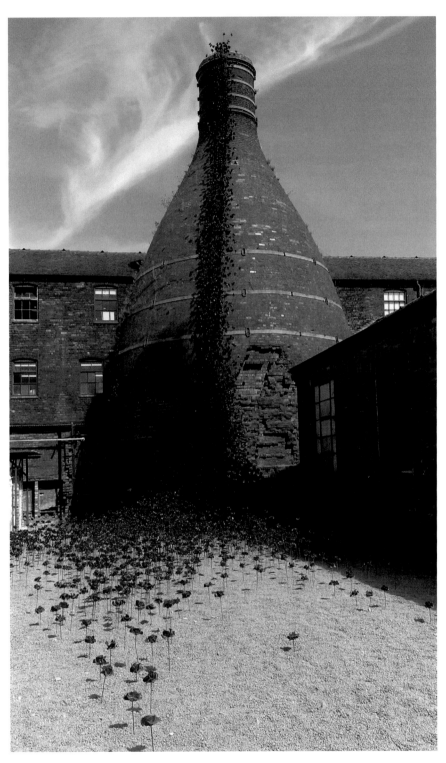

Middleport Pottery –
A Time Capsule of its Own
(Page 52)

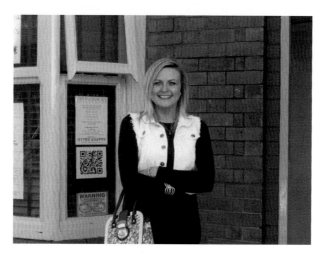

Blonde Bombshells of 1943: A Review
(Page 58)

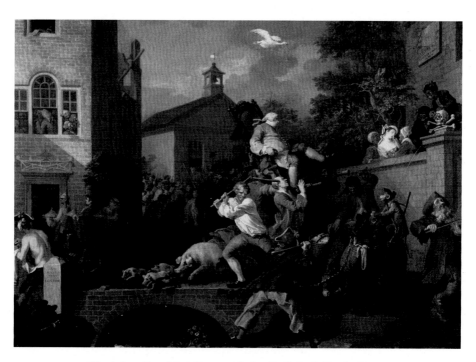

Chairing the Member and the Political Sixth Sense
(Page 85)

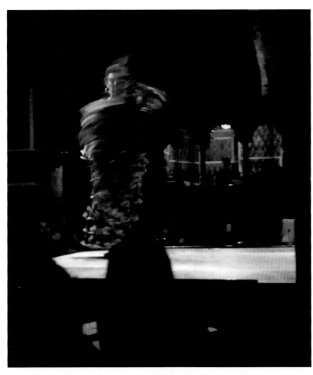

Imagine Liverpool's
John Lennon Airport
Accessible
(Page 87)

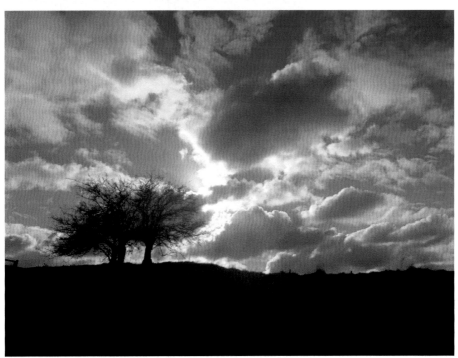

"Not Saxon but Celtic" say Experts
(Page 97)

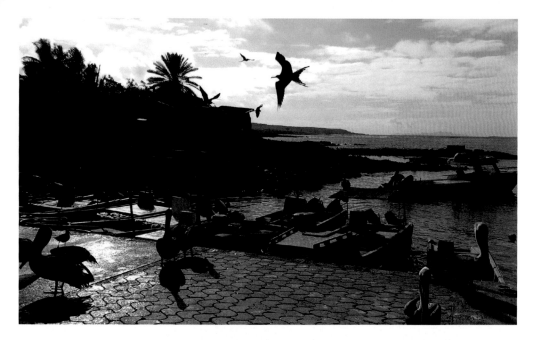

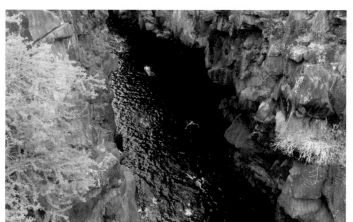

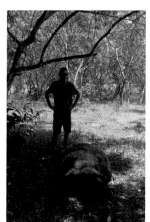

Galapagos: Islands that Time Forgot

(Page 69)

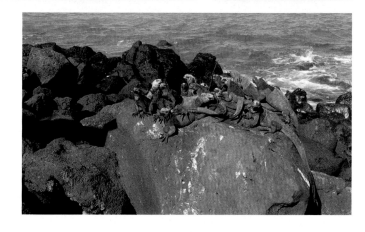

Galapagos: Islands that Time Forgot

(Page 69)

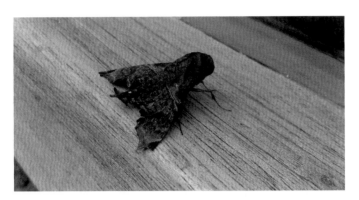

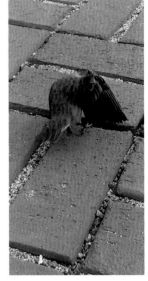

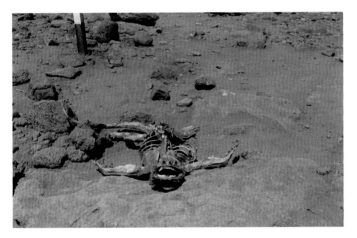

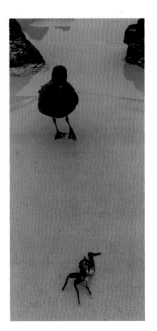

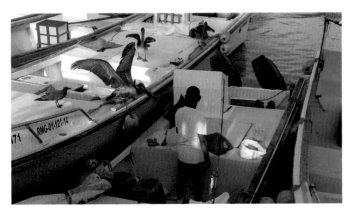

Little Pidge
(Page 104)

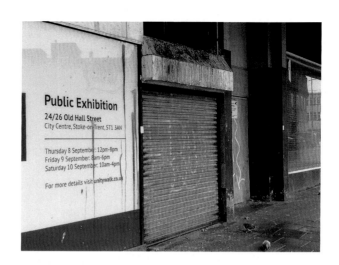

A Long Way from
Tipperary to
Newcastle for Sister
Agnes
(Page 119)

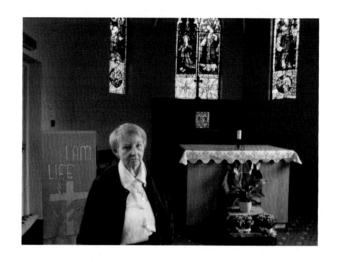

Inside O'Connor
series
(Page 134)

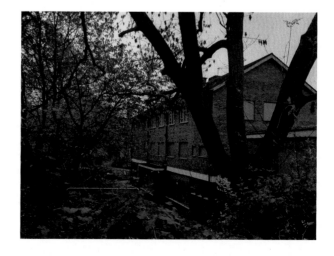

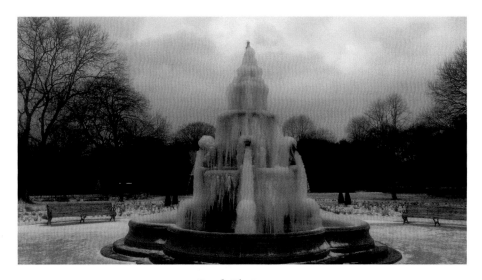

Cool Christmas
(Page 171)

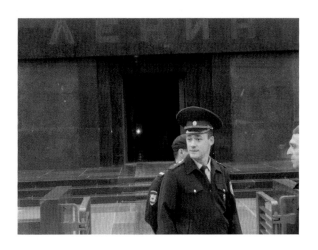

Dispelling those
Moscow Myths
(Page 180)

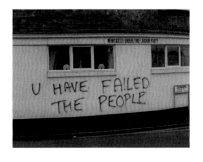

Extinction a Real Possibility
for the Labour Party in 2015
(Page 183)

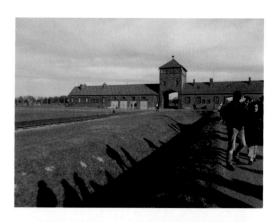

Auschwitz-Birkenau:
the Visitation
(Page 205)

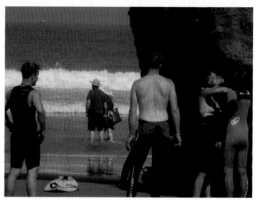

Basque in Biarritz, Anglet and
Bayonne for Half the Price
(Page 217)

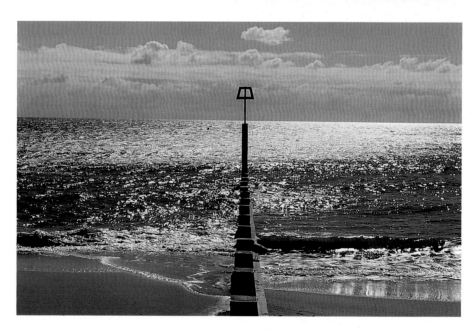

The Glorious Tattoo
(Page 229)

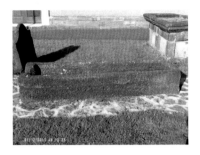

Seeing is Believing
(The Ghost of
Molly Leigh's Crow)
(Page 247)

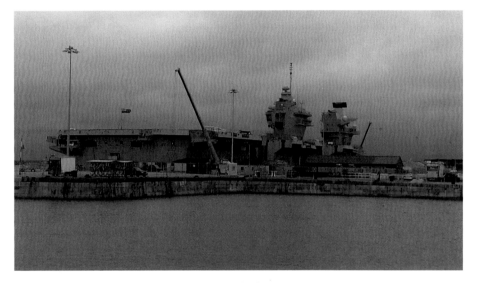

Naval Blue
(Page 257)

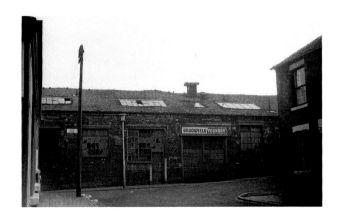

The Marl Hole
(Page 262)
Image courtesy
of Ken Cubley

The House on
Greenbank Road
(Page 289)

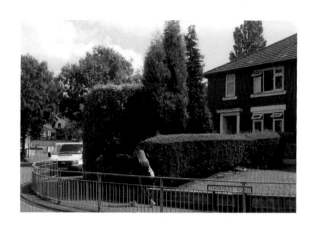

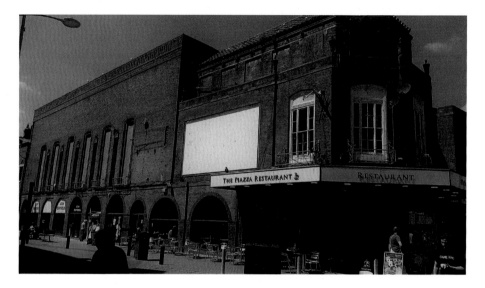

The Paper Cart
(Page 296)

The Romans were
Taking the Pee
(Page 323)

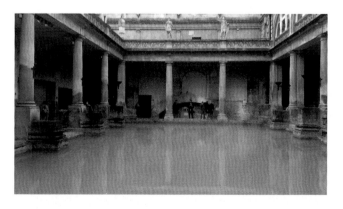

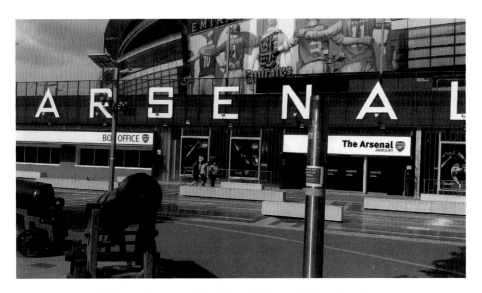

Rebranding our Stadia: A Bitter Pill to Swallow
(Page 344)

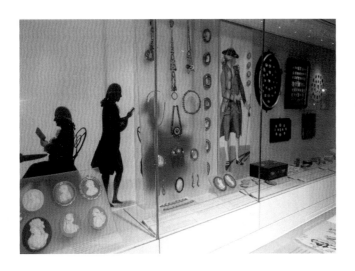

Demonstrations at
Wedgwood for
the Select Few
(Page 361)

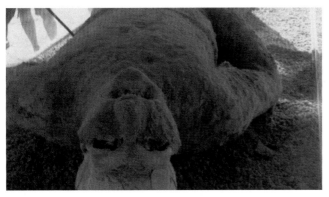

Pompeii 2011:
You Couldn't See
Me for Dust
(Page 365)

The Final Chapter

(Page 376)

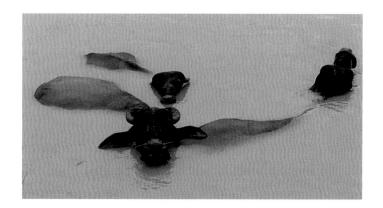

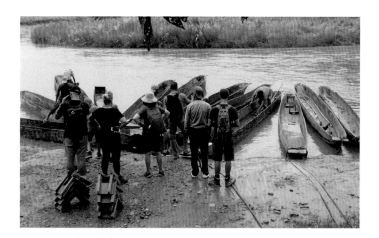

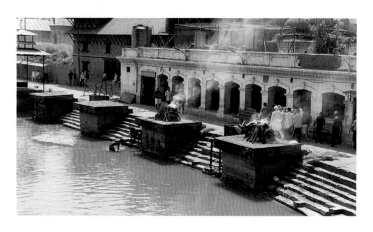

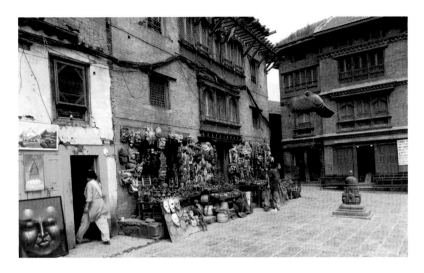

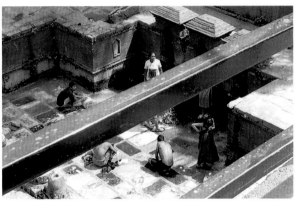

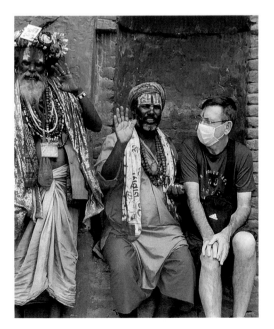

The Final Chapter
(Page 376)

The Final Chapter

(Page 376)

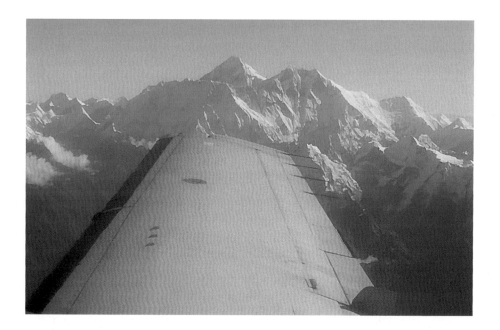

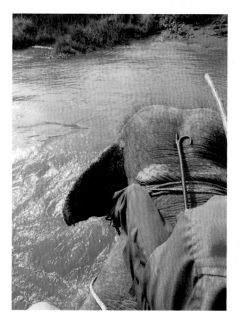

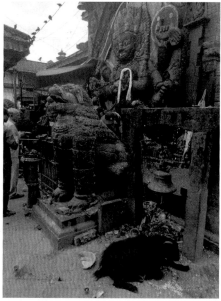

Sucky Blood in the Amazon Rainforest

I was lucky enough to visit Manaus in the Amazon rainforest in November 2010 which is 2,656 miles from Rio de Janeiro. I had also planned to spend a few days in Rio, before and after my trip to the Amazon.

Alarmingly, my flight luggage was lost/misplaced and while Air France were making enquiries in attempting to locate the baggage all I had was what I stood up in. The anxiety levels were to get a lot worse after two days being luggage-less. There was a shopping centre nearby in central Rio, but when I visited, my bank card became defunct when attempting to draw out cash. It was not the best of starts to my once in a lifetime South American experience. Then, just as I was about to have a nervous breakdown (after several locals had tried to assist me with my bankcard) Michael, who I had met previously in Galway, popped into mind. The same had happened in Galway with the same bank card and he had advised me to give the card a good wipe (or rub like you would Aladdin's lamp). I did just that, and there and then my card worked. The Real poured out. A few rags were then hastily bought for my expedition into the rainforest (opting for dark forest green and brown colours to accentuate the natural thread).

The first morning I awoke in my little cabin deep inside the jungle, largish-looking cockroaches were crawling on my face. This was the rainforest, it was reasoned, so it might be in my best interests to respect the biodiversity and become at one with the inhabitants, so I just scooped them off and got on with it. There was also a large-legged spider guarding the brown natural pool near to the lodge, but it was deciphered that it was the insect's territory, so I kept well away when dipping in. The natural spring water appeared brown but was in fact clear and when you moved around in it you would experience pockets of warmth due to the sun managing to shine through gaps in the dense trees. It was quite unusual.

One short night safari saw me meeting the large, odd, sort of sitting upright frogs, who would have appeared more at home in a Disney animation film. They made loud unusual croaking noises too. On another trip, I swung through the trees on a rope swing and got a bullseye from firing a dart from the blowpipe. Even the native tour guide was impressed and he could shimmy up trees like the lithe wild animals (he reckoned it was down to eating catfish – not exactly my speciality). Yes, Kev would have one of the best chances of surviving if push came to shove he determined, admiring the new T-shirt bought in haste from a Rio store. He had made it with no luggage, when others might have stammered and faltered facing the same unforeseen setback. Now, it seemed, he had even gleaned inside information in that Viagra was in fact made from rainforest tree extracts, which brought about a whole new meaning to the expression 'getting wood'.

After seeing the strange stick insects, which don't just look like twigs, they have the same consistency, and being acquainted with the bad-tempered parrot who had made his home at the camp, on a morning rainforest safari I was bitten by something strange. It was a sort of fly, the size of your average bluebottle. I actually declared that I had been bitten and so the tour guide caught what had bitten me red-handed (in mid-air would you believe in his bare hand) and so we all, including the Russians, the British (little ole me), the Belgians and of course the native Brazilian, huddled around to examine the specimen. The tour guide then held the flying creature by the wing and informed us that it was only a baby and it had 'sucky blood'. On interpretation, this meant that the cheeky scamp had taken my blood and if this was the baby, I would have hated to see mother.

To think, my blood is now indigenous to the Amazonian rainforest ecology, perhaps for all eternity.

On My JACO Jones

For those looking for redress after being spoken to disrespectfully by a judge, don't go to JACO (Judicial Appointments and Conduct Ombudsman).

At a civil hearing, I had never been so humiliated and insulted in all my life by the sitting judge. His personal 'charm', in how he spoke to not just me but the Clock representative and the barrister, casts a shadow on the whole judicial process. The judge was not just extremely rude; he was an odious, obnoxious blackguard.

When I reminded the judge that his manner was inappropriate, he threatened to have me removed from the court.

Beforehand, this judge had me running up to his desk with court papers inducing fear in a litigant acting in person – already perplexed with the elitist and establishmentarian legal stage. I then informed the judge that a complaint would be made against him and I did not want him to preside over any more hearings involving me. He replied that it's all on transcript (recorded), to which I stated that his tone should be on transcript too.

The judge in question also spoke dismissively to the shocked Clock representative but she opted to play down his behaviour by describing him as 'having a bad day'.

Anyhow, the two aforementioned, who were also present at the hearing, might suffer in silence in response to this kind of treatment just to further their careers, but I was having none of it, even though it was known deep down that my critical voice would be the lone voice. After making contemporaneous notes, JACO were then contacted so that the judge could be investigated forthwith. I also requested that any subsequent investigator should listen to his pugnacious tones themselves. In addition to his voice, his body language was also supercilious, especially when he told me to 'get out' of the courtroom (or words to that effect).

The judge's manner was commensurate with that of a bellicose bully. In fact, condescending arrogant dinosaur figures need to become a thing of the past if our legal system is to ever modernise for the benefit of all.

When initially dealing with a representative from JACO regarding my complaint against the judge, her manner was impatient over the telephone even though I obviously felt distressed and belittled. I made a statement in writing regarding her approach, which she said was down to being short-staffed.

I had requested that I should be able to listen to the recording featuring the judge, but of course this was out of the question. My complaint was then just closed down without any referral or explanation of the next step. The JACO rep said she had listened to the audio of the hearing and could find nothing wrong with the judge's conduct.

When I requested to be copied into JACO's correspondence to the judge when he was notified of the complaint against him, so I could gauge the character of the JACO address to those on high, it was said that a copy could only be provided for a fee.

When JACO then asked that current bog-standard question of what I wanted from the complaint, I replied that I was hoping (beyond hope) that those being complained about would be reprimanded and JACO would change accordingly from the elitist and snobbish organisation they are conveying themselves as. I went on to say that it would be productive if management at JACO made statements to the effect that they are going to change the culture of the organisation, and most importantly, they intend amending their policy of instantly jumping to the judge's side at every turn. I also stated that I would like the statistics regarding how many cases they have found in favour of the complainant (redacting names of course).

Psycho-architecturally

Psychological warfare is an interesting concept and my visit to Shrewsbury in October 2013 enabled me to engage with the curiosity. Whilst in the beautiful town, I noticed that Shropshire County Council was situated in an old Tudor building and this set me thinking about our own Stoke-on-Trent city council and their U-turn regarding their determination for staff to desert the fit-for-purposes civic offices in Stoke, for a new glass tower complete with rosy garden in the so-called central business district of Hanley (voted one of the worst buildings in England) costing millions of pounds of taxpayers' money. Remarkably, after all the consternation surrounding the Stoke move, Newcastle Borough Council announced that they were demolishing a beautiful Victorian school, built by our ancestors under difficult working conditions, to erect a fancy new house for themselves on that same site costing £15.4 million. They were also fully operational at the civic offices in Merrial Street. Aren't they the important ones?

Statements from the leader of Newcastle Borough Council regarding the school, such as, *"If you want to stay in the Victorian age that is fine and dandy but I do not"* are insulting. It's not about what career councillors want, but about local people wanting to retain their beautiful architectural heritage. All the council does is demolish one building to build another (Jubilee Baths for example), it's preposterous. Simultaneously, the only ideas proffered on how to spend our taxes is to finance shopping centres for multinational concerns who offer nothing but low-paid jobs. They say the new council HQ will be cost-effective. Well, let's add up the cost of demolition and rebuilding in Newcastle over the years and do a compare and contrast with utilising/replenishing existing Victorian architecture over the next ten years shall we?

The original civic building in Merrial Street, the old library and the Guildhall are now empty (November 2018). And annoyingly, the councils new 'one stop shop' HQ forces members of the public to address private matters like benefits at a counter, come library, come public space.

With regard to the city council, admittedly, the U-turn was not an unequivocal surrender, as they still built their unwanted 'Little House on the Prairie' at taxpayers' expense, albeit in an age of austerity. But the council's new decision to keep council staff active in the civic building in Stoke (obviously swayed because of local anger) was almost tantamount to a truce of sorts.

Back to Shrewsbury, but still talking amnesties; amidst the dreamy spires decorating the tranquil banks of the River Severn from the standpoint of the English Bridge; it appeared that there is a military significance permeating the town.

We have the infamous battlefield dating from 1403, located some three miles north of Shrewsbury, which is one of only forty-three battlefield sites in England and Wales. Addedly, on the way down to Shrewsbury from Newcastle/Hanley, one can see modern military compounds like RAF Shawbury and Tern Hill near Market Drayton, which also adds to the military experience.

On doing a U-Turn (just like the council) to the initial point in question: it does not need a long, psychological battle to convey the message that the architectural aesthetics that adorn Shrewsbury's every corner are down to one simple manoeuvre.

There is no point in erecting new buildings at the expense of demolishing the old ones. Stoke-on-Trent City/Newcastle-under-Lyme Borough Council take note; intelligence gathering is cost-effective in avoiding a dirty campaign of demolition.

Less than Equal

The vote on legalising same-sex marriage in Ireland in 2015 was a monumental milestone in Irish political history. What is more, the outcome was decided by a national referendum (the world's first) which initiated a change in the Irish Constitution. In other words, the notion that those God-fearing relics in the outback of rural Ireland would say five Hail Mary's at the mere thought of a same-sex union were nothing but idle myth.

Ireland irrevocably changed by social revolution; except for those six little backward counties in the north whose bigoted factionist Unionist overseers (the DUP) oppose equality even though the UK establishment they don't want to be different from, has adopted same-sex marriage accordingly.

In the resulting celebrations at Dublin Castle one young lady epitomised the meaning of the result when stating that she was not 'less than' for being gay (or words to that effect). Over the centuries there are other prejudices, myths and stereotypes associated with Ireland to cement painful suppressive feelings of being less than. In that throughout the centuries and even in my generation, perennial propagation purporting that the Irish are perhaps 'a little thick' which took the form of subtle Irish jokes and suchlike, implanted the notion in the home country's population that the Irish were an inferior race and were treated as such.

This has led to conflict.

Note: I did hear one English joke (the only one I have ever heard) when I lived in Dublin. Nonetheless, I was quick to point out to the teller that I was English, so I wasn't impressed. Yes, I was lucky I didn't get a clatter (a Dublin expression for getting a slap).

Turning back to subtle indoctrination, the Anglo-Irish zeitgeist over the years saw the Irish being typecast as 'ginger-haired', Papist and/or subversive. In fact, the red hair physicality was brought over to these islands by the Vikings (Scandinavia). Predominantly the Irish are dark-haired by natural design (there is delicate Spanish influence in some ports like Galway).

Neither the Anglo-Saxons nor the Romans ever colonised Ireland.

More recently, we have been party to the Irish immigration nonsense where in England the Irish have been portrayed as immigrants by leading politicians such as Shadow Home Secretary (2018) Diane Abbott to back up Labour's pro-immigration stance. The reminder being from Ms Abbott that not so long ago, England's job advertisements were accompanied by 'No Irish need apply'. Yes, this was the case, but it does not back up their wider argument regarding immigration in that they maintain Irish Citizens in England are on the same par as African/Asian immigrants. Can you leave the Irish out of your immigration party politics in future please? You know as much about this subject as Secretary of State for Northern Ireland Karen Bradley (2018) knows about Northern Ireland. Or better still, read up on British geo genetics a little more profoundly. The Northern Irish (some being Irish citizens not UK citizens) are officially classed as being part of the UK.

The Irish cannot be immigrants on their own islands (the British Islands) as I will explain. Although my nationality is English, culturally I am half (or even a quarter) Irish and although both cultures have merged genetically, one cultural side can predominate the other at different intervals and eras determined by external and environmental factors.

Existentially, in the home nations, if we are white, we are most likely to be English, Scottish, Welsh, Irish, or a British islands mix. The Scottish, Irish, Welsh and English have all implanted their genes in each other's lands (the Irish even invaded Wales, would you believe, many moons ago).

Therefore, taking into account the English and Scottish plantations in Ireland over the centuries, do we call the Scottish or English descendants of those plantations (who then become Irish) 'descendants of immigrants'; of course we don't. In addition, do we also refer to Scottish settlers in England as immigrants?

Yet again it is just the Irish that are singled out and made to feel less by those who should know better.

Despite the fact that on the British islands, the English, Scottish, Welsh and Irish have always had free movement (one does not need a passport to visit Ireland from Britain and vice versa) politically, there is a need to assert our independent constitutional identities in relation to which home nation we owe our allegiance.

Some refer to this phenomenon as nationalism.

Whatever the terminology, culturally and racially, the statelets on these islands will always be genetically linked.

The Institutional
Name-Changing Game

On the 15th August 2017, I was both devastated and shocked at the response from the South Cheshire Clinical Commissioning Group regarding a Stage 1 Dispute meeting, where a decision was made to not award my mother CHC (Continuing Health Care), taking into account just a couple of weeks after the CHC review in question, and as a result of being forcibly removed from her care home, she died. For those not familiar with CHC, it is when the NHS rightly provide the nursing care because there is a health need. The alternative is that the person's savings will be decimated and their house sold to pay for that same care.

The like institutions (commissioning groups, for example) all play their part in the death of vulnerable older people in one way or another; they are in fact complicit in the decisions being made on high that are bringing about the death of people before their time. Not to mention the appalling NHS care they preside over, like the CHC reviews, which impose further indignity and distress on already grieving relatives. I really don't know what sort of people they are; can anyone else out there ascribe appropriate descriptors?

I was ordered by this particular commissioning group to go straight to IRP (Independent Review Panel) when, through their incompetence, I was not notified of the Stage 1 Dispute meeting because the person presiding over the case had left. The group maintains that they did not receive any written communication from me, when it clearly says in a letter written on the 17th January 2017 from the former employee that a colleague would contact me to set a date for the Stage 1 Dispute meeting. No colleague contacted me (maybe because the employee had already left the organisation); which was the reason why I telephoned the number in Nantwich some six months later to ask why I had not been contacted.

Is it therefore fair to say that the 'team' are manipulating distraught family members and in essence, making it up as they go along when placing a charge on people's houses.

This sham of an institution has even changed its name from Restitution, Complaints and Disputes Team to Appeals and Retrospective Review Team, to further confuse and frustrate anguished families.

Institutional name changing is the oldest one in the book.

Tickled to be in Europe

The continental weather we had been witnessing in September 2011 of twenty-five degrees befitted the fact that Stoke City were playing in Europe again. Was, therefore, the sun about to shine on Stoke's Group E match against Turkish side Besiktas? The supporters' pre-match activities saw some of the 1,700 Besiktas fans strolling around Hanley clad in coats and scarves, would you believe (being used to forty degree temperatures in Turkey must have made our sultry late summer seem cold).

Home fans were also in the strolling mood and were tickled pink to be in Europe. One such fan realised one did not have to be in Essex to experience the new fish pedicure priced at £5 for twenty minutes located in Hanley's Tontine Street. It would be a tonic to soothe those pre-match nerves. Yes, the only way is up Anley duck and one quickly concluded that the Stoke fans are as cultured and civilised as any other on mainland Europe.

One noticed that in one tank there were smaller 'tiddler'-like fish and in another, there were bigger fish and when one asked the Chinese assistant what the difference was; she replied, "You can have little tickle or big tickle." I opted for ten minutes of a little tickle with the smaller fish, to be followed by ten minutes with the bigger ones, and yes, it was a rib-tickling experience, fish nibbling at your feet.

On to the match itself. In the early exchanges Besiktas took the game to Stoke with some clever midfield play orchestrated mostly by the number four, Fernandes. Besiktas' Portuguese number seven, Ricardo Quaresma, was a class act and his imaginative passing split the Stoke defence on more than one occasion. In contrast, Stoke were chasing shadows, exemplified by Whitehead who looked below par even though Stoke had made seven changes to the side that had drawn with Manchester United. It was no shock then when Besiktas went into the lead in the fourteenth minute when Quaresma slotted a fine ball into the path of Hilbert, who scored with a low shot to the bottom corner.

Stoke replied immediately with a corner from Whitehead. Shawcross's shot was blocked, but Crouch was there to stick his Daddy Long Leg out to force the ball over the line. This seemed to be the only clear-cut chance for Stoke in the first half as they struggled to play football at ground level.

Half-time: Stoke City 1 Besiktas 1.

Not being able to get a ticket for the Manchester United game, it was wondered when the deft flick-ons by Crouch were going to materialise as espoused by some Stoke fans who had been at that game. Then one mused whether Crouchy needed the feet-tickling treatment on his shooting foot as one of his shots skewed well wide in the latter stages of the second half. Talking of tickling, the Besiktas goalie Recber was hardly tickled by the Stoke forwards, but dramatically collapsed in a heap on more than one occasion. Some of the continental sides might play the game to the delight of the football connoisseur, but to the football cynic, the play-acting contradicted any quality football they may or may not be capable of delivering. When the weary Etherington went off for the lively Pennant on fifty-one, and with Walters replacing Jerome on fifty-nine, the game seemed to turn in Stoke's favour after a shot by Quaresma had deflected off Huth and hit the post. Walters was troublesome going forward and the Turkish goalie did well to tip his shot onto the woodwork midway through the second half. Stoke stole the game on seventy-eight when another corner saw Crouch impeded by Sivok in the box and Walters made no mistake from the spot.

At the outset of this competition, Stoke City were 80/1 to win the Europa League. Perhaps the benchmark to measuring how far the club has progressed is seeing that after the Besiktas game; they became 20/1 to lift that same trophy.

Full-time: Stoke City 2 Besiktas 1.

Attendance: 23,551.

Court in the Act: a Titillating Tragedy

I called into Stoke-on-Trent County Court (which doubles as a crown court) on the 26th February 2018, for what one would term 'advice', not knowing that yours truly would be the one who would end up in the dock. There was an evacuation of the courts so we all went outside (including the judges). I took a few snaps of the milling crowds because, being a writer, one always needs an image to fit an article. I knew the laws regarding taking photographs but was not aware of the law with regard to court precincts. I did not think for an instant there was any wrongdoing. I stood on a public pavement while I took the photographs which can be evidenced.

A judge was recognised exiting the court building because he was stupid enough to allow his flashing purple robes to be seen under a long dark coat. This was lax security.

On my return to the building, I was shocked to be ganged up on by a 'hench man-like' security team who started to threaten and bully me, stating with words to the effect that a prominent judge had complained that he was not happy with someone taking photographs outside. It crossed my mind at this point in time that the security guards fancied themselves as police officers themselves. One security guard threatened that photographs had been taken of him personally, which was not the case. He also held on to my phone because it had gone through security X-ray, which he had no right to do.

I then requested the police be called (as the situation had become so alarming) so they could examine the photographs. One of the security guards then disappeared inside the court.

A plain-clothed police officer was then brought down from an upstairs court and I showed him the images. He then 'just walked off' after perusing them. By this action, in him not deleting the images or arresting me, it was assumed that there was no case to answer.

The drama then continued, with me by now in the metaphorical witness box (the court foyer) answering a barrage of questions from the court manager and of course standing my ground. Yes, there was a commotion. The manager was told countless times when she asked to see the images that a police officer had already viewed them. This official responded by saying that she had a responsibility to inform the police (or words to that effect) regarding the photographs, which disturbed me even further.

It seems odd that the judges don't like the idea of photographs being taken of them (because of security issues). One doesn't suppose those guilty of a felony savour having their photos taken by the photographers of local papers, who hover outside court snapping impecunious individuals on entrance. An offender's face in the local paper is more than a security issue; it ruins what life they have left. Most of the offenders being photographed have mental health issues/addiction problems and are already feeling very low. Being photographed and further humiliated in the local paper cements the notion in the offender's mind that they are 'undesirables', so more often than not, they behave like undesirables and offend once again and so the criminal cycle continues unabated.

When newspapers promote tragic cases in their low-brow publications and describe the characters in the stories as sub-human 'thugs' or 'drug addicts' it does not depict the whole, sometimes vulnerable, picture or past personal histories of the offenders in question. This, in turn, convinces the public reading the stories that the paper is doing a public service. It can be argued that many local papers are doing the public a disservice because crime rates are climbing. Can we therefore state with conviction that some journals are ruthlessly profiteering from tragic titillation? What is more, are national and local rags alike, at best, putting a lid on the offending epidemic, and at worst, putting the public in greater jeopardy? Newspapers should not be in the position to affect crime rates.

The system in place needs to change – it is not working. Just look at the statistics regarding the escalation of crime, drugs (including alcohol) and mental health problems. Therefore, those guilty of some types of offences should not have their photographs taken and splashed all over the local paper. They need to atone for their crimes, seek help and then be able to move on to become a valuable member of society; not to consistently reoffend, as is now the ingrained pattern.

Turning back to the incident in question, after returning home, I waited for the police to call to take me in for interrogation, which was very upsetting.

I later did some research and found that, according to Channel 4 News:

"Filming parties to proceedings as they arrive and leave the courthouse is also technically forbidden but in practice this rule is not enforced; e.g., pictures of defendants and witnesses arriving and leaving the Royal Courts of Justice or the Old Bailey are commonly shown."

Newspapers regularly photograph people on the concourse of crown court precincts, so could someone please answer why they are flagrantly allowed to break the law and take photographs of those with mental health/addiction problems? What's more, the moral question should be answered as to why the powers that be allow newspapers to illegally take photographs to be published in the local paper, which by all accounts contributes to, and makes worse, the offender's already humiliated mindset. Obviously, they are then more likely to reoffend.

Note: this matter could not be clarified with the Ombudsman because Paul Farrelly MP, refused to refer the case.

Auschwitz-Birkenau: the Visitation

It was a poignant but troubled experience visiting the Memorial Museum of Auschwitz-Birkenau, the biggest of the Nazi German concentrations camps constructed during the Second World War. It was not what one would term an Elysian experience, knowing that 1.1 million people had been exterminated in this notorious death camp, a statistic which would disturb the most balanced and unemotional amongst us. Just a bus journey from Krakow in South West Poland, the site is not to be overlooked, especially if one wants to grapple with comprehending what human beings are capable of and the underpinnings that expedite such brutal wickedness.

Ideas that the extermination of the prisoners is fallacious is an absurdity in itself.

On the bus from Krakow, I could not help but note the forested area and pondered if some of those being taken to the concentration camps in the years 1940–45, via the same route, would have had the same view. How must they have felt?

Costing just a few pounds, it is wise to have a guided tour of the camp and don't be afraid to ask searching, but respectful, questions; I most certainly did. We want to know exactly what went on (like the sinister medical experiments carried out by Clauberg and Horst Schumann, who researched a convenient mass means of sterilisation). We can only begin to understand the horror of what happened on the premise of knowing the full facts.

What stood out during the visit to Auschwitz was learning about the Factionaries, who were the most brutish and sadistic German convicts, brought in to the camp specifically to terrorise the camp population. For myself, I am usually absorbed in psychological peculiarities, such as the fine line between that of civility and baseness in the human condition, which would determine me analysing what some detainees would inflict on fellow detainees, to survive themselves.

I saw where Rudolf Höss, commandant of the death camps, was hanged in 1947 and detected his family home nearby. In the 1940s it must have been very strange how normal family life co-existed in an illogical oasis amongst the carnage of terror. I also viewed photographs of what appeared like male detainees, but in reality were female. All human identity, including female identity, had been systematically stripped away from those interned. I also observed a display of tons of human hair which was used for mattresses and stuff, but visitors were not allowed to photograph this exhibition.

The postcard hoax, to me, was the most revealing during the visit to Auschwitz-Birkenau. In a glass case, postcards sent from Jewish detainees in Auschwitz to relatives all over Europe are kept. Of course the prisoners in Auschwitz were forced to write the postcards and were dead via the gas chambers before their relatives received them. The postcards, dictated by the Nazis, would stipulate to the relative that at Auschwitz they were well looked after, well fed and the work was light. Word spread and those facing persecution in their respective countries could not wait to get to Auschwitz. Greek Jews paid for their own tickets and spent a week in the cattle trucks getting to the camps.

I had asked the tour guide at Birkenau (a short bus ride from Auschwitz) why, after the gruelling cattle truck ride, where many suffocated on the way, did the passengers not become suspicious of what was awaiting them? I had answered my own question, in that all they had was hope. In addition, why would the migrants not believe what their relatives had told them about Auschwitz via the postcards?

Yes, it was scheming of the most disconcerting kind on behalf of the Nazis.

For me, what needs deeper analysis regarding this important historical period in Europe is why the majority of ordinary people, just like you and me, were complicit in the demonisation/extermination of the Jews. Why were Jews detested so much within their respective milieu and what or who was the conductor that facilitated anti-Semitism to enable such a holocaust to prevail?

It is thought that Polish priests and nuns were also sent to concentration camps like Auschwitz because they were thought to have much influence on society. They did not survive long because they would not beg, steal and scavenge like the lay internees.

Footnote: all 15,000 Soviet (Russian) captives perished at Auschwitz-Birkenau.

The Accent on Period Drama

Set in the five towns in the years beginning 1872, *Clayhanger*, by Arnold Bennett, is one of the very few filmic pieces to be set in the Stoke-on-Trent area. No sex, drugs, violence, expletives or American characters; simply *Clayhanger*.

Made by ATV in 1976, *Clayhanger* is a watchable tale set in Bursley (Burslem) in the late 1900s. The twenty-six-episode story ambles along nicely where the acting gradually improves to inform the viewer of the love between Edwin Clayhanger (Peter McEnery) and Hilda Lessways (Janet Suzman). Although not in the same league as *Upstairs Downstairs* (which depicted the lives of the lower classes as well as the middle and upper) *Clayhanger* does harbour authenticity. Some of the props and settings seem to exude poignancy especially to those from the Potteries area (with help from our local museums). It seems almost possible to make out Market Passage in Burslem (off Market Place adjacent to the present Leopard public house).

A clever touch for this dramatisation is that before each episode an authentic introductory synopsis ensues, whereby a voice informs us in one sentence the essence of the previous episode and the one to come, which points to theme originality. On the other hand, it takes a few episodes and the first part of another before the *Clayhanger* family trope switches to Tunstall (Turnhill) in a somewhat abrupt manner, focusing entirely on the Lessways, which confuses the viewer to some degree. *Clayhanger* struggles at times, especially when some episodes dramatise the two-person setting, which to some is appealing but to others is mundane.

The portrayal of the Potteries accent in this series is quite laughable. Received Pronunciation (RP) dominates, as do Brummie accents, Yorkshire accents, a bit of Lancashire and a touch of East Midlands. It appears every twang is audible but for our own Potteries accent (with the exception of the opening episode 'Last of a Schoolboy', wherein a young messenger boy briefly informs the young Edwin to convene at the Dragons Hotel). One knows the accent is difficult to emulate but good actors after spending time in the area should be talented enough to grasp its dialectic variations. The dialogue throughout the series is lightly peppered with local sayings such as 'please thee sen' but because of the lack of working-class characters, these expressions are often spoken by the middle classes, which, in turn, asks the question, would the middle classes have spoken in that fashion?

Man: Made for Disaster

While staying in London, I decided to visit the burnt-out shell of the Grenfell Tower, where some seventy-two died in the still unexplained 'great fire' of London. The fatality figure is still a contentious issue, taking into consideration subletting and illegals that could have possibly been residing at the tower.

Latimer Road tube station was closed, so to get to the tower I had to go via Shepherd's Bush. It's not morbid to visit and one does not have to feign grief. To see for oneself the blackened tomb that was once people's homes, one can perhaps begin to understand the malicious forces that are endemic in our society, orchestrated by our controllers who preside over that same system. I observed that the media were still there, and although the story had largely faded due to the cyclical nature of the media circus, investigations are still ongoing. Personally speaking, social housing generically should be analysed during any investigation which would uncover the correlation between social housing landlords not listening to their tenants and the possible catastrophe that can ensue because they turn that deaf ear.

Back to the media, who should definitely be brought into focus regarding this tragedy. Are they not just puppets to their billionaire establishment masters who will just about photograph, film or record anything or anyone for money? Then we have those so-called 'journalists' who demonise those who espouse fairness and accountability as Marxists. This is no more than sinister. Oh sorry, I forgot; it's their job, isn't it?

I took many photographs of the Grenfell area and was concerned when a police officer came over and said very nicely that some residents might take offence because I was taking photographs. I replied that I was not taking selfies; as in bunching around for group photos with the burnt-out tower used as some kind of warped backdrop. There are always those who like to pull rank, aren't there? As many photos should be taken as possible of this grotesque monstrosity, to demonstrate a reminder regarding the state of Britain in 2017. Then people can post those said photos on social media to politicise this abomination. That's the only way things will change.

I don't know what others think, but what I find extremely annoying is when political figures are asked a searching question on man-made disasters like Grenfell, they always say something like, "First let me give my deepest sympathies to the families and my thanks to the heroic emergency services." Is this a delaying tactic? As in, was this response learnt at 'Spin School'? Just answer the question I say and forget the platitudes. The tragedy has happened and you did little to prevent it. This idea suggested by the fire service for residents to be sitting ducks in the event of a fire and stay in their flat is ludicrously dangerous. In all fire situations, you get out if you can. You would not know what started the fire, or if other fires are about to start. Not to mention explosions. The fire service propagates one predictable set of rules for evacuation, when, by nature, fires are extremely unpredictable.

I recall taking legitimate fire concerns right to the top of the complaints system with a social landlord some ten years ago, where it ended in court. The fire service officials at that time were dogmatic, bureaucratic and ignorant and did nothing but blag/cajole at every opportunity. I can call to mind one occasion when an unprofessional fire service representative responded to my contradictory evacuation assertions with the juvenile phrase of: "Listen here, sunshine."

They also colluded with the Housing Association being complained about as already discussed in a previous article. Nonetheless, this point needs making again.

Back to Grenfell, alongside the tower could be seen the 'relief effort' which occurred after the tragedy had unfolded. It reminded more of a jumble sale.

This so-called relief effort was not even properly coordinated by the incogitant Calamity Jane (Theresa May) and Co. Perhaps Calamity was so busy cosying up to the DUP gunslingers who are supposed to be riding shotgun to this government farce, that she probably didn't note the magnitude of the disaster.

A thought occurred when I saw a beautiful little chapel across from the Grenfell Tower. Perhaps the so-called Christians in the Conservative Party, the Tory-Lites in the Labour Party and the Lib Dems in the Finished Party should visit and bow their heads in shame in the hope that 'God' will forgive them.

I certainly wouldn't. They allowed cost-cutting profiteering at the expense of safety.

A Little Pressure
Sometimes Pays Off

In 2012, it was a colossal battle to get to the truth, even regarding something as simple as the future of the former Maxims and Zanzibar nightclubs, which were eyesores in a smart Newcastle-under-Lyme town centre. Newcastle Borough council has only now faced up to the problems posed by Maxims and the Zanzibar, when previously they hoped the problem would just go away. After contacting the council early in July regarding the fact that Zanzibar was a dangerous structure, the Deputy Development Control Manager at the council said:

"The former Zanzibar building is not a listed building and is not considered to be a dangerous structure. It is understood that this building is being marketed and periodically enquiries are made as to the development potential of this site."

Regarding Maxims, she went on to say:

"Whilst a conditions survey has been undertaken which identified that works were required to the building, the council has not stated that these must be done prior to the sale of the building. The owner is presently arranging a secure fence to be put around the whole site to prevent access to what is a potentially dangerous structure. I would recommend that you contact the owner of the building to ask the question regarding what works have been undertaken."

When I suggested that they sounded like they were afraid to contact the owner of Maxims and that taxpayers are paying staff at the council to do the contacting, the Head of Planning and Development took the reins and rapidly changed tack. He said:

"*With respect to the Zanzibar there have been further developments which my colleague could not have been aware of when she wrote to you on the 5th July. The Building Control Partnership (between the City Council and the Borough Council) received reports of an allegedly dangerous timber plywood canopy on that day, the site was visited, the situation was deemed to be dangerous and following unsuccessful attempts to contact agents who had acted on behalf of the owner of this property in the past, the Partnership arranged for works to be undertaken to make the situation safe and these works were then undertaken.*"

Sort of getting warmer, weren't we?

Abracadabra: today, in 2018, both structures have been completely revamped.

The Second-Hand Shop Towns

All across the country and on every High Street, second-hand shops have sprouted up, with merchandise now featuring price tags just like major stores.

Talk about a recession.

Stoke town has been dubbed our second-hand shop town due to the number of charity shops in the once thriving civic centre. On Church Street alone there is more than a handful.

One can go so far as to say that Stoke has become a commercial shell following Americanised ideas of mall-like shopping centres exemplified by Festival Park, coupled of course by personal financial restrictions in that 'nobody's got nowt'.

Typified by a mix of second-hand shops and run down empty business premises, Stoke has fast become a ghost town in dire need of investment.

On Glebe Street healthy businesses can be unfortunate enough to have derelict premises sandwiched in between them.

Beside, the once famous 'Harry's Bar' has become non-operational after years of being the nightlife beacon and hub of the town, but that is perhaps due to the change in drinking habits, which is another article.

It seems a travesty that prosperous businesses can be penalised for being adjacent to derelict buildings. Surely, new legislation is the answer; building owners have a duty of care in respect to their neighbours.

As for second-hand shops; many like to have a mooch around in them so they must serve a purpose, even if some even sell second-hand underwear.

The Inquisitive Wild Boar

Wild Boar rummaged through the leaves on the even wilder
forest floor: he thought that the trees were all made of draw

Yes he sniffed all day from dawn till dusk
From that little nosey inquisitive tusk

Rummaging here and sniffling there
Little did he know it would be death for a dare

Curiosity perished the boar. Legs stiff in the air.

Wild Boar had been mooching home one dark night

Weird Wolf was of narcotic, alcohol and sprite
Temptations aplenty wild boar should have took flight

Boar swigged at methylated liqueur; thought he could take
the pace. Avarice for more, addiction took place

He collapsed forthwith no time for Wolf to lace. Alcohol
danger he had completely lost his face

Hell on this earth he was as white like a ghost
Wild Boar ending up as wild boar roast

Mixing Greed had overcome and death had adorned

Had inspired substance gluttony, Weird Wolf was not mourned.

Basque in Biarritz, Anglet and Bayonne for Half the Price

The Basque trio of Biarritz, Anglet and Bayonne (all less than three miles apart) in south-west France (Pyrenees–Atlantiques) can be visited via flights from Britain which are not overly expensive.

Sun seekers (with temperatures scaling 38 degrees in September), culture vultures and surfing enthusiasts alike can all carve themselves out a four-day summer break that just about has it all. Yes, the south of France can be expensive but like my mum used to say, "You cut your garment according to your cloth."

If one is going to cry oneself to sleep after pretending to be loaded (thus paying £8 for a diet coke in a flashy bar instead of shopping at supermarkets) then perhaps one should stick to the Costas. Besides, the patisseries (bakeries) offer a mean floury/sugary snack at a reasonable price.

Remember over 90% of the inhabitants in the south of France are on similar budgets as us (well maybe that's a little exaggerated) so just be yourself if you want to blend in and go unnoticed. Talking of which, a polite "*bonjour*" when using French services should suffice, remembering that most French people that can speak English will do so to seize the opportunity to practise. Sprinkle in a little French of your own intermittently if you do engage in conversation, to let them know we are not completely 'language dumb' in old Blighty.

Eventually, and after a couple of days, you may even be mistakenly assumed to be a French citizen yourself (like I always am). This does not mean you have to guzzle their coffee, of course. The best advice is take a little travel kettle and your preferred choice of tea or coffee. Cafés in the area will charge nearly £3 for half a cup of lukewarm 'American' coffee or their own little pot of 'black ink'.

If you want to get about in the region the bus service Chronoplus can shuttle you between Biarritz, Anglet, Bayonne and the airport for a single euro or so fare.

The main beach area in Biarritz perches astride the vast Atlantic Ocean on the Spanish border and is a lively holiday destination attracting a mix of ages (mainly French). Apparently, the height and velocity of the waves make it an ideal surfing area. In contrast, the beaches in Anglet are a little more reserved than your Biarritz counterpart. This does not detract from the natural beauty in abundance though.

The main attraction in the old streets of Bayonne is the Basque Museum where artefacts of the Basque culture are well set out in this modern airy building. The entrance fee is six euro (2012) and the exhibits (including the brilliant Fandango portrait) are not explained in English so you have to utilise your French and work the significance out yourself.

Now that's an education.

What About Those in Care Homes Who Have No One?

When Heathside House care home closed down in 2011, Stoke-on-Trent City Council maintained that there were other facilities to accommodate the elderly, many of whom were suffering from dementia (there were care issues with regard to my mother who resided at Heathside House that are documented).

What the council did not inform was that the homes available were out of county – in Shropshire and Cheshire.

Initially, my mum was housed at a local facility but since falling fourteen times at that care home the management instructed Stoke-on-Trent City Council that they could not cater for her and would produce a legal document to remove my mother if the council didn't.

My mother was eventually placed at a care home the other side of Church Lawton, Cheshire, with the only other alternative being a very run-down home in Shropshire. When I couldn't get a lift to the home it took me one and a half hours there and the same time coming back. I also had to walk for a thirty-minute stretch through lack of public transport to the home.

When farming the old and the vulnerable out like this it means that they have less chance of visitors because of the distance to travel. When I couldn't get a lift to the home it took me one and a half hours to get there and took the same amount of time coming back.

Late in 2014, I had two or three telephone calls informing me that my mother had fallen out of bed. I eventually contacted the occupational therapists from East Cheshire Council and reported the matter to the CQC (Care Quality Commission).

Cheshire East Council mitigated that there were other priorities and it would be a few weeks before the occupational therapists could assess my mother. I could not think of a higher priority than a very frail eighty-year-old lady on an end of life care plan with advanced dementia who was allowed to keep falling out of bed. Her legs had also begun to lock in the foetal position. Whoever heard of a dying woman falling out of bed?

When I eventually met with the occupational therapists on October 16th 2014, I felt as though it was three against one (the two occupational therapists and the senior care worker). During this meeting they deflected my points instead of addressing them.

This was exemplified by the more vociferous of the occupational therapists who responded that my mother was not seriously hurt when she fell out of bed the last time.

I replied by expanding on the distress and psychological damage incurred; my mum shrieked when cold hands were put on her but the therapist did not seem to understand or show any compassion.

One of the occupational therapists then mitigated that there was a new bed that had come out which could be placed on the floor. I then stated that I had requested something like this months ago but really all that was needed was that mattresses should be aligned to where my mum was positioned, so if she fell out she would roll onto the mattresses and although it would be distressing for her she would not injure herself. I accepted that rails either side of my mum's bed could cause her to become entangled.

The therapist then asked me if I could fund this new bed, to which I said no. The quieter of the two therapists then intervened and said my mum would qualify for the bed because of the care package she was receiving. They could not tell me how long my mum would have to wait for this new bed. I concluded that if my mum should fall out of bed again the situation would become very serious.

I stated that I only have another person's word for it that every time my mum has fallen out of bed it has been documented.

In other words, in the real world, one can never be entirely sure that every time someone had fallen out of bed the incident had been recorded, so in effect, she could have fallen out many times.

The more vocal occupational therapist declared twice in relation to addressing the problem that 'she would do this for me'. I responded by saying that she was not doing it for me but for my mother.

I then contacted the health care body in Staffordshire that was supposed to be overseeing my mother's care. A representative went out to the home and reported to me that everything was fine.

It took some months for the new bed to arrive and even longer for the mattresses to be aligned to guard against her falling out again.

Then at lunchtime on Thursday, July 30th 2015, I was aghast to see food caked thickly all around my mum's mouth. It was not just a little bit, but spread over a large area. I told the care worker feeding my mum that I was not happy as it looked like he had been shovelling the food in. The care worker responded by saying that he cannot help it if food gets around her mouth.

When you witness something like this alarm bells start to ring.

I then went to see the manager to report this matter as this was about my dignity and my mother's dignity (which should have been covered in basic care training).

It was also mentioned to the manager that every time I visit there is a different agency staff worker on duty. It was also put to her whether or not the home is aware of the theory regarding the benefits of continuity of carers for those with dementia. To my knowledge some seven regular staff had also left in the last few months. Many professionals would concur that if staff members start to leave in any given job it suggests that the workplace is not a constructive or positive environment to be in. The reasons are usually because those staff are overworked, ill-used and paid little. Extremely ill and vulnerable people have to live in this environment that is not fit for well and able-bodied people to operate in so what does this say about the care home in question in the wider context?

Later that day, the situation became even more distressing after I read a newspaper article highlighting that same care home. There had been an investigation by the CQC. The investigation had been carried out in May and still little had changed at the facility even though a new manager had been brought in to resolve the inadequacies. The situation was about to get worse when I contacted the CQC who gave me the link to the scathing fourteen-page report on the home. Some would argue that the neglect identified in the report is commensurate with abuse. The Health and Social Care Act had been breached some thirteen times.

I also contacted the emergency social care team at Stoke but they failed to respond.

As an addendum, all I can say regarding our care home system in England is that this current profit-making culture coupled with cuts to basic services augurs the question as to what the situation will be like when it comes to our turn to be admitted. If some believe money will save them they could be in for a nasty shock.

It appears there are some good care/nursing homes out there (where the owner invests in patient care) but they are a minority. The majority of care homes are production line establishments where to capitalise from the vulnerable adult is the main incentive. You cannot profiteer from dementia care because by doing so one would have to streamline one's costs which in turn could only be reduced by cutting the quality of care. In effect, the care home dysfunctional cycle evolves as follows. When neglect, abuse and/or degrading treatment occurs to a resident in a care home, the relative/friend/overseer inform the CQC as is their right. The CQC then contact the council to request a safeguarding review. The council via a social worker then go to the home to air the relative's grievance and the home either denies the charges or states that they will do A, B or C to address the problem usually after a safeguarding meeting with relatives. Then something else untoward (or even the same thing) occurs again and so we go through exactly the same process again but are back to square one because nothing has changed.

If the proprietors of care home establishments dare to allow this level of care to those who have family members overseeing that appalling care, where does that leave the unfortunate souls who have no one?

Thinking Inside the Box

He appeared confused as he permeated the idea of the deep wound gurgling dark maroon. He did not want to die; not yet anyhow. Not in this fashion. Not on his own with nobody to assist with the transition from this sphere to the next.

Open but sceptical to the concept of gods and religions it brought no comfort; he still said a prayer though. Atheism was not the issue here; death was. The figure was going to pass painfully, alone – painfully – then nothing.

The man could inform that there had been nothing but there had, when he got there, but there wasn't anything but nothing, there that is.

The Compartmentalised
Matchbox

Scant breathe, no more ears and wax
Compartmentalised, no – not going to Cockney Rhyme to
say one's gasping for cracks
Of sulphur spreads noxious to my microscopic nose
How, why the cylindrically square container-tox-ious
Noxious plume give me air – not prose
This is not Kafka's 'Metamorphosis', this is real life socio-
confinement
Compartmentalised and entombed in life's denouement

Crackhouse Reborn

I was ejaculated with a groan and guttural grunt under the influence of *Scrumpy Jack* and crack cocaine.

He was so much more emaciated, smaller, weedier, more discoloured and smellier than the uniform man.

"Can you lend me 20p?" he had whined with that smack-head accent outside the pound shop just hours before the event.

I am now larger and almost have a heart.

There's a knock at the flat door, another scally? What's the betting the word script is uttered in the forthcoming garble and yes that word gear?

I can smell their Primark rags from here; yes to be embellied is rather queer.

That puddled Lindy has just emerged and when she loses it, well you ain't seen nothing like the ruffian scraps she involves in. Probably over a quid.

Will little unformed me survive the ensuing skirmish and filthy carousel?

Well here's to hope – hoping I'm terminated.

You could have Blown me Down with a Feather

Myself and other residents were at our wits' end regarding twenty-year-old outdated and dangerous fixtures and fittings in properties supplied by the social housing provider. Just like the housing association at Grenfell Tower, they refuse to engage in a positive manner and for the most part they both penny-pinch and/or ignore the issues raised. The antiquated heating system (it was a refrigerator that started the Grenfell fire) where your electricity bill doubles when using them go cold at around 8pm. Other residents will attest to this where a petition had already been signed. I was shuttled through the Housing Ombudsman process regarding the heaters; who took two years to respond. Then the Ombudsman took the side of the provider and appeared to be in their pocket. Not so long ago, housing associations employed ordinary token housing association residents as ventriloquist dummies to frustrate the complainant even further. The Housing Ombudsman, in my experience, is just another line of defence for the institution complained about. Regarding the Ombudsman generally, even if they find for you, there has be an injustice. In many cases, there is a prerequisite that your MP must refer you to the Ombudsman or your case cannot be heard at all; how discriminatory is that? This means that if a privileged self-serving cog of the system (which is mostly the case) does not get on side, your complaint cannot even proceed.

On July 15th 2017, the twenty-year-old door to my bedroom jammed. Which begged the question what would have happened in the event of a fire? What if the door had jammed when I attempted evacuation? It then took two twenty-minute phone calls to emergency, who replied that workmen would be out sometime that day.

I had also struggled to open the catch on the windows. The workmen could open them because they were familiar with the catches but I must say that when I tried it was very difficult, with or without problem hands – it's a tricky manoeuvre. How the elderly, vulnerable and the disabled are supposed to open these catches, especially in the event of a fire, only God knows. In this case, the workmen put oil on the catches because they were so stiff, therefore this begs the question: should this not be cyclical, as in checking fixtures and fittings which could, in the event of a fire, be a possible escape route. I have since discovered that the window frames are wooden and the housing association don't fit wooden frames anymore because of fire concerns. Wood burns, you know.

Apparently, the workmen could only come out regarding my windows within a six-hour time frame (12–6). I had to wait in until 4pm for the workmen to arrive after having an assurance that they would come nearer 12 (there are also reports that this social landlord treats their workforce as poorly as they treat their tenants).

I also noted that the chief executive of the housing association does not respond; is he too busy to address tenants? You know the ones, the ordinary people who finance inflated salaries.

Residents had already stated that they would meet with representatives including political representatives, the social landlord and the fire service (who do not seem to have a clear-cut policy on evacuation, but some kind of bog standard generic outline, as all ready explained). Conversely, we said we would like the materials used to build our homes checked for flammability, considering that as a company the landlord behaves like a mean spirited Dickensian hock shop where every attempt at redress for legitimate customer concerns turns into a stressful battle.

To conclude, I thought I would relay this true story. I called the same housing association some five or so years back because the cheap windows and frames were letting in cold air and in the winter months, the bedroom was becoming really cold (the living room had been fitted with a second glass shutter behind the main windows to insulate against the draught). Even though I bought blinds and heavy velvet curtains to insulate against the cold in the bedroom it was still no deterrent and after I complained, two officials came out, both suited and booted. The male agent then proceeded to drop a feather from the top of the window frame to the bottom of the sill to demonstrate there was no draught.

I told him to get out.

This is the mentality those who dwell in social housing are up against.

Note: in the autumn of 2018, residents received correspondence stating that new doors and windows were to be fitted on properties at the complex. Yes, they eventually caved – probably because of Grenfell Tower.

The Glorious Tattoo

It appears that the recent hot and sunny spells seen in England in July 2013 and throughout the summer of 2018 was not to everyone's taste. We are not used to the heat.

Furthermore, according to 'weather forecasters' there is more to come. Could we possibly, in future, bear witness to much more of that spectacular consecutive fifteen days of summertime as experienced in 1976? Regarding the summer of 2018, although the sunny days were not always consecutive like that of '76, the summer was overall, the best I can ever remember. During past summers, the marginal battle between the clouds and the sun always saw the clouds win through. In 2018 it was the sun's turn to shine. The sun fought the clouds and the sun won.

When the sun is scorching, older people especially are more at risk from dehydration and exhaustion, while others of all ages hope and pray the heat wave will end very soon because, well, it's just stifling (and that's without the humidity).

Sunny dispositions matching the sunny weather do not always correspond. Irritability, lack of patience, tetchiness and even anger can surface when out and about especially when travelling on non-air-conditioned transport. Let me tell you, the bus experience during hot weather is tantamount to torture.

Then we have the 'insect invasion', where strange creepy crawlies appear from nowhere. Let alone the abundance of those pesky (or should I say dangerous) bluebottles, house flies and midges (in size descending order). Notwithstanding, in the summer of 2018 aggressive bloodsucking horseflies were also frustrated with the heat; they bit hard and infected fast.

Still, the prospect of brighter days sees calm mood and serotonin levels rise, especially with the younger generation who cannot seem to wait for that first glimmer. Stripping down to the bare essentials (supposedly because of the heat) seems to be the order of the day and who can blame them; they have been covering up from the cold for most of their lives.

There also seems to be ongoing an unofficial competition regarding the person who sports the most novel tattoo (my personal favourite is the Christ the Redeemer statue in Rio de Janeiro, especially when encompassing the shoulder to the spine).

Then we have the water experiences; it's nice to be beside the sea, rivers and streams in the blistering heat, where many can experience the delights of activities in this sphere without freezing to death.

It's funny how we change as we get older though. In your twenties you would have sold your soul for just a week of glorious sunshine. Now it seems for some, the relentless days of beautiful weather are tolerated grudgingly.

To end on a high, on a visit to Dorset in September 2018, I witnessed the summer closing in. Having seen countless seas and oceans around the world; none was as spectacular as the English Channel on that day, sparkling from the late summer sun (see centre pages).

Amsterdam by
Ian McEwan: Review

Son of a sergeant-major, Ian McEwan with *Amsterdam* (1998) offers us a snapshot of archetypal London life in the middle and upper professional classes during the 1990s. To say it has come under critical spotlight in literary circles since winning the Booker Prize is perhaps putting it mildly.

The narrative opens describing the life of Molly Lane, quintessentially a restaurant critic, who has just died, aged forty-six, having suffered a terminal disease. At Molly's funeral, her husband George and former lovers, all in the throes of middlescence, have gathered to pay their last respects. One of those former lovers is composer Clive Linley, another is newspaper editor Vernon Halliday, and last but not least, Foreign Secretary Julian Garmony got in on the act as another aficionado. As one usually does at funerals, Linley asks his old chum Halliday to euthanise him if he should ever fall irreparably ill. Halliday agrees to do so just as long as Linley agrees to return the favour – and so the plot begins to somehow gain momentum around the two main characters, Linley and Halliday, told in third-person narration.

The opening pages of *Amsterdam* discuss the bickerings involving the three warring men (Linley, Halliday and Garmony), with McEwan, through Clive Linley, jibing at the pretentiousness of the monied classes including those amongst the funeral congregation. This can be illustrated when Beat Poet, Pullman, is ridiculed quite colourfully as: "A withered little lizard of a man who was having trouble twisting his neck to look up at Clive." McEwan also uses Linley to make a political point when Linley looks around at fellow mourners to cynically add how they had all flourished under a Conservative government they had despised for seventeen years. "When the ladder crumbled behind them, when the state withdrew her tit and became a scold, they were already safe, they consolidated, and settled down forming this or that – taste, opinion, fortunes."

Consequently, *Amsterdam* then morphs into a Halliday vs Garmony (press vs politician – privacy vs morality) tale – photographs of Foreign Secretary Julian Garmony are discovered by George Lane (husband of Molly) depicting Garmony dressed in women's clothing. George, the husband and puppeteer, pulling the strings of his three love rivals, promptly sells the photos to newspaper boss Halliday who is editor of the publication *The Judge*. It must be said that crossdressing is hardly a newly revealed oddity for the curious reader to wince over. For this particular crossdresser to be a Tory foreign secretary aspiring to be PM is hardly salacious either; the political classes are not immune from sexual impropriety or 'difference' just because of their standing.

The significance of the support female characters and bit part players, Molly and Rose, in McEwan's second novel is not fully understood. Although Molly features in the story line she has already died a slow and agonising death. Some would argue that although deceased, Molly presents as the main character, immortalised as a liberal minded sort of upper crust good time girl, thus influencing the narrative from the outset.

Rose, wife of Garmony, on the other hand, is characterised as the loyal, strong wife of the transvestite coxcomb who faces the media with a strength and self-confidence not commensurate with embattled downtrodden stereotypical wifey types.

As *Amsterdam* unrolls, we are forced to endure Linley's stream of consciousness of his tortured mind and it's at this point that the reader begins to tire. We are then subjected to Clive Linley's visit to the Lake District for him to gain a much needed fillip for his next musical masterpiece. Then, oddly enough, another innocuous moral question arises juxtaposing scenic landscape this time around. This moral dilemma concentrates on Linley choosing to abscond and concentrate on his melody rather than to intervene in helping a woman engaged in a violent fracas with a man.

The storyline pans out in a similar vein as the novel progresses, where Linley muses on finishing his musical masterpiece. Alcoholism appears to surface at this interval, where McEwan, through Linley, takes us around his posh abode simultaneously cursing Halliday in a sort of squiffy cerebral monologue where the word genius is liberally banded around (the genius tag ascribing to Beethoven and others, not Linley). To wrap up this section of the account, Linley then duly appears to suffer from a bout of alcohol-induced cerebellar ataxia and flakes out.

The euthanasia or assisted suicide undercurrent begins to take shape within the narrative during this part of the script, with the now bitter enemies, Clive Linley and Vernon Halliday, negotiating their final assignation and possible termination. The conclusion centres on Amsterdam which, together with Switzerland, are construed as the assisted suicide capitals of Europe.

Without spoiling the lacklustre twist to this very mediocre text; let's just say it was a dull end embroidered by the karma influence.

Not all would agree with the lacklustre and mediocre analysis though. Douglas Hurd, the former British foreign secretary who served on the panel of judges, deemed *Amsterdam* a sort of wise examination of the morals and culture of our time.

Whose morals and whose culture, one might question?

Analysis

Wooden third-person narrative dimmed by the dull/pretentious lives of the middle and upper classes.

Amsterdam Condensed [Book] by Ian McEwan is published by Vintage Paperback
178 pages
ISBN 0099272776
Topic: Book Reviews (Fiction)

No Mug's Game

When leaving school at sixteen, I embarked upon a work experience programme as a catering assistant at the Royal Alexandra Hospital in Rhyl, where I received the grand sum of £21 per week. You were expected to work weekends too. I complained to the boss, my excuse being I could not travel from Rhyl to Stoke-on-Trent to watch Stoke City on a Saturday afternoon, so I was transferred to the Prince Edward War Memorial Hospital (PEWM) down the road. It was a joy to go to work at the PEWM (not as slave driven) and I had my weekends free too.

At school, most of the pupils had supported Liverpool as they were the dominant club in English football throughout the late 1970s. I did make the point that most of those in my year supported the winning team, and as such, two school friends began to support Wolverhampton Wanderers instead. We would alternate between watching Stoke City and Wolves. On one occasion in 1978, we even travelled as far as London (White Hart Lane) to see a Division 1 match between Tottenham Hotspur and Wolverhampton Wanderers. My favourite fixture of all time was the match played on the 3rd March 1979, between Stoke City and West Ham United. Stoke won 2-0 in this their promotion year. West Ham brought a big, interesting mob and were marched down from Stoke station (under the bridge) to the old Victoria Ground where Stoke City played their home games.

I had told my school friends that as a child I had visited the Victoria Ground on many occasions. This was not the case; I became seriously interested in Stoke City as a sixteen-year-old and my first game was Stoke vs Burnley in 1978. I had only visited the ground once before and that was because a teacher from St Peters Junior School took me and a classmate to the stadium on a weekday to meet the players. I recall that my mate had a fancy autograph book, but I had to ask (Jimmy Greenhoff, Alan Hudson or Denis Smith – I can't recall which) to sign my blue-lined A4 page, I think they provided the pen too. I wasn't really interested in cherishing signatures, even as a ten year old.

The match between Wolves and Everton at Molineux in February 1979 is distinctly recalled. This was because on the way back from the match a group of Everton fans burst into our train compartment to rough us up. The phrase 'Woolly Backs' which meant we were not from the Liverpool area, was uttered. I felt hands going all through my pockets and later my mate declared that he had lost his wages, him being on leave from the Merchant Navy. We notified the train guard who contacted the police, who then boarded the train at the next station. The police then took me into a toilet cubicle with one Toffees fan who I had recognised, and my mate went into another cubicle with another officer and fan that he had recalled. I was shocked when the police officer ordered the teenager to strip right there in front of me; underpants and all.

The most revealing story regarding supporting Stoke City from North Wales was when a group of us went to Blackpool and we all bought a mug with our favourite team emblazoned on the side. I then decided that a good game to play on the train home was to fill our mugs up with water and throw it at people through the window as the train pulled out (yes, it was disgraceful behaviour).

At Chester, I threw a mug of water over a guy as the train pulled out; I was shocked to the core though when he got back onto the train. Overcome with fear, I looked at my friends and when they turned their heads to look out of the window I knew I was on my own. Swept by terror, face ashen with fright, I ran down the train, still holding my Stoke mug, which was by now incriminating me due to the evident water droplets still cascading down the side.

When the very angry man caught me he gave me a clip around the earhole; I got off lightly. He must have travelled a long distance out of his way to teach me a lesson I would never forget.

The build-up to the season saw Stoke City vying for promotion back to the top league and it all rested on winning at Notts County on the last day of the 1978–79 season (May 5th 1979). Popular songs in the charts were *Wow*, Kate Bush (17), *Jimmy Jimmy*, the Undertones (28) and *Goodnight Tonight*,

Wings (5). A sea of Stoke fans amassed the visitor enclosure at Meadow Lane for the match between the two oldest clubs in the football league. Stoke went on to win 0-1, thus sealing promotion back to the big time. On the train home to Rhyl, I can reminisce seeing a local paper broadsheet which headlined: *Stoke win and go up.*

The season had ended in more ways than one; just four weeks later we would move back to Stoke-on-Trent from Rhyl permanently.

Food Vouchers for Benefits: You can Bank on It

As benefits are cut, more and more people have to rely on food banks. Some would say that the argument for replacing benefit monies with food vouchers is already in operation. If the benefit is cut, then one has to rely on free food vouchers to survive. Furthermore, the government is becoming increasingly reliant on food banks to deliver food to the hungry in our communities. This is in light of the fact that one of the most demeaning things a human being will ever do in their lifetime is to beg for food.

But more and more are discovering that they have no choice – especially if they have young and hungry mouths to feed. There are prerequisites for access to the free food, as in one has to be referred from local agencies (made up of medical practices, housing associations, DWP, CAB and schools – as in those on free school meals).

It must be said that many agencies defer their decision on whether to issue the vouchers and others, like the DWP and the county/city councils, have strict means testing rules before they will issue a voucher that will enable people to access food (like a benefits suspension), in that these agencies have to tick the reason specified on the food voucher as to why the person is in need before food can be despatched.

Many would make the point that every day is an emergency for those living on benefits or living on a low income.

In some cases the food can be dropped off. But more than likely the one applying for food aid will have to visit the food bank centres at certain times to be allocated nourishment. When one requests a referral from one of the participating agencies they can only be issued with three food vouchers in any one crisis. For a single person, one food voucher can provide food for a three-day period. If the crisis then escalates beyond this nine-day limit one has to return to the referrer for a further assessment with no guarantee that vouchers will be issued again (as of 2013).

The food given in exchange for the voucher has been assessed by nutritionists and is thought to be a healthy balance.

You could have fooled me. If starvation doesn't kill those facing pecuniary shortfalls, the fatty, processed, sugary food on offer at the food banks will.

Remembering 1914-18 for all the Right Reasons

With the centenary of the First World War occurring in 2014, the lack of understanding from the established order has seen them not quite knowing whether to troop out in their worst black cloaks or their best party frocks. This is because most of our so-called dignitaries aren't quite sure whether the 100-year anniversary of the Great War of 1914–18 is a sombre occasion or one to celebrate.

According to the British prime minister at the time, David Cameron, in a speech at the Imperial War Museum, he advocated that the great massacres should be remembered with a: "Commemoration like the Diamond Jubilee celebrations which says something about who we are as a people."

Sixteen million people were expunged and a further twenty million were wounded during this bloody and brutal conflict where our young men (and women) were used by the ruling elite as expendable resources in an eerie selfish game mutating into entrenched warfare.

Hardly merits Diamond Jubilee-like street parties, does it?

It can be argued that to quietly remember the actions of the brave, young, innocent but powerless military personnel is a much more fitting accolade to those that made the ultimate sacrifice.

It is thought the First World War was instigated by three royal warring first cousins (all grandchildren of Queen Victoria) and their pursuit of imperial power in Europe at the turn of the 20th century. During this era, the British Empire ruled a quarter of the world and massive profits were made from the colonies.

There was King George V of Britain, Kaiser Wilhelm II of Germany and Tsar Nicholas II of Russia all vying for supremacy in the prelude to war, where Britain formed an uneasy alliance with Russia and France against the enemy axis of Germany, Austria-Hungary and Turkey. Ironically, even though Russia's royal family (the Romanovs) were related to George V and Russia was an ally, they were still refused entry to Britain during the Bolshevik Revolution of 1917.

Close on one million Britons (including those from the Commonwealth) were butchered because of this regal dispute and 130,000 were slaughtered on all sides in one single battle, that of Gallipoli.

Yes, there are parallel subplot theories to contradict the three cousins' rationale as to why the First World War was instituted. Nonetheless, if the aristocratic directive wasn't the catalyst for starting the fourteen–eighteen war, what other reasons have wars been fought for over the centuries if not for wealth, power and territory?

This notion should be the linchpin for Remembrance in 2014–18. Lest we forget; the masses will never be ill-used in privileged power-hungry war games by the ruling classes ever again.

Six Feet Under Scores
the Best of US film

Usually preferring the realism of British scripts, it must be said that when the Americans do engage in reality, whether it be fact or fiction, they do so well. *Six Feet Under*, which ran from 2001–05 and featured sixty-three episodes, underscores the gritty drama US style, focusing on the fractious and dysfunctional Californian Fisher family who run a funeral home in Los Angeles. If one saw the series the first time around it is a definite must to view it again, such are the sophisticated storyline plots projected through the dark and sinister backdrop of death. Nate (Peter Krause) plays the brother everybody would love to have and his brother David, played by Michael C. Hall, is cast as a semi-closeted gay man and patriarchal figure of the family. The opening episode features the death of the father, Richard Jenkins, (Nathaniel Fisher Senior who then, in turn, reappears throughout the series). The mother (Ruth Fisher) played by Frances Conroy, also plays a good part and was nominated for Outstanding Lead Actress in the Primetime Emmy Awards.

Written by several writers including Alan Ball, Rick Cleveland and Kate Robin, *Six Feet Under* was nominated for numerous awards and deserves its place as one of the greats. The series' opening music, composed by Thomas Newman, also won an Emmy in 2002 for Outstanding Main Title Theme Music. Although the music sets the tone for the darkly original plots to unfold, the series is not characterised by stories of gloom and doom. Human relationships and dilemmas (and the emotions that go with it) often present, which can invoke a sense of empathy for the viewer. Some of the actors, including Lauren Ambrose (Claire Fisher) and Rachel Griffiths (Brenda Chenowith), genuinely aggravate the viewer, which must in itself be professional type-casting.

What sets the series apart is the novel way all of the episodes start with a death, which reinforces the notion to the viewer of how random and simple one's demise can be. Although fiction, the series relies on facts regarding the after-effects of death post-mortem, (a little bit of tautology there) including the strange peculiarity called priapism.

It is not in the pipeline to resurrect or reinvent *Six Feet Under*, as in dust it off and bring it back from the annals of classic film, as seen with other classics (which have been tarnished as a result).

Although now deceased, it is not forgotten.

Psychoanalysing London-Centric:
A True Story

To psychoanalyse a huge sprawling metropolis like London, we must examine not just the mindset of the inhabitants who spend time there but the maladroit governing institutions which are London-centric by nature. Although a multiculturally diverse city, there are still people aplenty who are afraid to challenge or speak out with regard to the mechanisms which control them. By contrast, I have never had a problem with challenging those who laud over us. In fact, I have written a true autobiographical account called *Hiding Behind the Institutions* which documents real-life courtroom dramas, such as when the city council's housing department was cross-examined on oath by yours truly and as such, one city council witness's neck turned a dappled crimson directly as a result of telling porky pies.

One distinctly recalls the judge saying, 'Okay, Mr Raftery, that's enough.'

This research starts on the train journey from Stoke-on-Trent to London Euston. For the time being let's not dwell on the raging pollution and backward/idiotic multiple omnibus system that all but paralyses the city of London and the multiple herds of human animals milling around, some in a dream-like state marvelling at our poisoned sights, and others en route to serving their masters in one way or another.

It appears that in August, 2017, the new ruling imposed by our comptrollers is to inflict the cold air treatment which occurs on trains, in hotels, in theatres and even in cinemas. Apparently, the powers that be deem that in August the hoi polloi, at intervals, need cold blasts of air sprayed on them because it's 'summertime'. Any oaf can tell them that in August our climate is not particularly clement and can be damp, cold and unforgiving. Air conditioning is only best served when the temperature exceeds 23 degrees.

Virgin Trains thought it wise to make the journey from Stoke to London as uncomfortable as possible with their spontaneous icy blasts of cold air. London Midland then obliged on the return with their brand of discomfort by subjecting me to prolonged cold spurts. What is more, even the Noel Coward Theatre in Leicester Square, which you would have thought would know better, ceremoniously spoiled the superlative *Half a Sixpence* experience (an interesting rags-to-riches English tale) by subjecting me to the cold air treatment during the 7.30pm sitting when the temperature outside was only some 15 degrees. When raising the matter before curtain call, I was told to "Shh" then ushered to a new seat a few rows up which was just as bitter. There is nothing one finds more irritating than to be told to "Shh". They were fortunate I was not a typecast ruffian, where a mild fracas could have ensued with me being dragged out of the auditorium in a headlock, all ruffled and dishevelled-like. Yes, I could have shown the performing middle classes, acting as the lower classes, just how to show one's arse. Instead, ninety minutes was enough, so I vacated at the interval, savouring my bit part by stroking my arms while theatrically murmuring "Brrr" in likewise simile.

You see the psychology behind the Cold Air Conditioning occurrence is that those in control cannot even be bothered to regulate the heating for us on a daily basis, as detailed to the ticket checker on the return journey, when I had asked him if the cold air treatment was compulsory. He had explained that some people complain it is too hot and the air conditioning is regulated at the depot. I replied that I had dressed for a 16–20 degree temperature (factoring in the fluctuation between North Staffordshire and South London) and had not considered the chill factor on trains. The ticket collector/checker knew he was well beaten because he didn't even ask to look at my ticket and yes, nowadays, there may be multitudes of barriers at every train station but there is no barrier to the repeated ticket inspection imposed on the public. It was therefore refreshing when a young lady in an adjacent seat backed me up by stating that she too was cold, or words to that effect. I and my new-found comrade, who had also dared to speak out, then discussed the thinking as to why the English as a rule don't make their feelings known, and why some appear uncomfortable or even annoyed when others do. I deduced that perhaps, in the subconscious, many are not comfortable with what they perceive as their masters being challenged because that would upset their belief system in the institutions that govern them, the reason being that deep down, they harbour a nagging doubt that in reality, those same governing institutions cannot be trusted, period. The young lady explained that having spent time in Germany and Austria it is the norm to speak out if things are not quite right and the majority are forthright in doing so. One wonders therefore if there is an interconnection between this and Germany's economic mettle/our economic anaemia.

There was no air conditioning problem at the Millwall FC café in South East London. Exiting the train at South Bermondsey around 9am to visit the stadium, I could not help but wonder if, in the old days, the Millwall fans used to wait around the corner of those steps to ambush the fearful visitors on match days.

The reason for the visit to Millwall FC was because I wanted to see first-hand how real, non-stereotypical Londoners go about their business. The Millwall Memorial Garden was also thought-provoking in that there was a sign advising against fans emptying loved ones' ashes into the garden and that they must seek permission first. This perhaps explains how much local football clubs mean to local communities, so those on £100,000 per week take note – stop taking out and try to learn to put back in. For footballers' wives to pay £40,000 for a handbag is offensive to the majority of ordinary people.

From south to north and on to the Freud Museum in North London, costing £4 with concessions for entry – the museum was in fact once Sigmund Freud's home. To be frank, although Freud was an Austrian Jew and was forced to flee by the Nazis in 1938, I could not help but wonder how he secured such a grand/beautiful home in leafy Hampstead complete with garden, but that's the cynic in me. Apparently, Freud was a trifle embarrassed regarding all the grandeur himself after living and treating his patients from a modest second-floor apartment in Vienna.

Although Freud only lived the last year of his life in the house off Finchley Road, it is a definite plus to have had such a notable psychoanalyst take residence. Inside the house a sign invited the visitor to lie on Freud's couch and engage with free association. Not being backward at coming forward I most certainly obliged and oddly enough, nothing came to mind, which was therapy in itself, although on a second sitting (or second lying) the Amazon sprang to mind (and I don't mean that money-grabbing US poor customer relations company). More seriously, it is thought that today we display objects around our homes just like Freud did to reflect our true feelings. These objects can manifest as toys. Freud reckoned that as children we can play with toys to deal with anxiety.

Talking of anxiety/disarray and to concentrate on the thrust of the article (the Englishman's or woman's psyche in that they are afraid to complain when subjected to shoddy service), at the hotel in King's Cross where I was staying, workmen were renovating, which was not declared before I booked. Although the hotel had generically followed suit with like institutions in setting the cold air conditioning accordingly (I had remedied that myself by asking for a heater in my room), at checkout I politely requested the contact details of head office, explaining that I had not been notified of the works being carried out, which was, in essence, misleading the customer. Expecting my grievance not to fructify and to be met by the usual objectionables, which would then turn into a polemic battle of minds, the lady on reception asked instead what she could do to remedy the situation. Taken aback, it was stated oh so very courteously that, "one or two nights' free accommodation would only suffice" but she instead refunded the fee in full for my two-night stay.

I vacated the hotel sort of smirking and later gave the hotel a favourable review. Yes, some would argue that I am guilty of self-serving and this is true to an extent. As human beings we are all egotistical by design, but in this situation to self-serve was to serve the majority. Whereas, if our controllers are forced to change their policies with regard to how they treat people just because of one individual raising an issue (note I don't use the word complaint) then as a society we all benefit.

One muses as to what Freud would have made of it all.

Psychoanalysis Definition

A system of psychological theory and therapy which aims to treat mental disorders by investigating the interaction of conscious and unconscious elements in the mind and bringing repressed fears and conflicts into the conscious mind by techniques such as dream interpretation and free association.

Seeing is Believing (The Ghost of Molly Leigh's Crow)

During Halloween (thought to be linked to an ancient Celtic festival called Samhain) one's thoughts turn to all things supernatural and ghostly. Burslem (the mother town of Stoke-on-Trent) has its own infamous folklore which was fascinating when growing up. The tale of the witch of Burslem, Molly Leigh (1685–1746) and her pet crow will live on in local history indefinitely. Molly was thought to have walked around the town with the bird perched on her shoulder. Then, when she died in 1746, it is thought that Molly Leigh, from the beyond the grave, sent back her crow to sit and squawk on the sign of the Turk's Head pub in the town to turn the ale sour.

Such was the hysteria then gripping Burslem townsfolk, that Molly was putting spells on the town via her feathery friend, the local clerics exhumed her body and buried her north to south which was at a slight right angle to the other graves in the churchyard. Before reburial, the drunken mob wickedly tossed her crow and best friend into the coffin still alive.

The last squawk was thought to be heard around sunset.

Could that really be the spectre of Molly's pet crow seen next to her gravestone? (see image in centre pages). Molly's pet raven/crow plays a significant part in the legend, where the bird is her only friend and companion in a community that Molly is ostracised from. In addition, did Ms Leigh have any family members, such as parents?

It is also believed that a 20th century witch, Sybil Leek, who claimed to be a descendant of Leigh's, also took to keeping a crow as a companion, just like Molly.

Was Molly really a necromancer, or just an eccentric loner who never quite fitted in? People could be cruel, especially in those days. Those that are different in our communities can be characterised as such (in Molly's case a sorcerer) which can in turn push them even further into the void of solitary isolation, where for many, there is no return. In effect, perhaps Molly started to display a weird comportment because she was characterised as such.

I can recall that as kids we visited Molly Leigh's grave in St. John's Churchyard in Burslem. We used to chime, "Molly Leigh, Molly Leigh, chase me up the apple tree," (not chase me around the apple tree as ascribed by some) three times, after which she was supposed to appear. Even though it must have been over forty years ago I can still recall that, disappointingly, Molly never did materialise.

British Classics Revisited

It was not because I took a module called British Television Drama while undertaking a degree in Media Studies that I found great interest in the 1960s British working-class film genre. In my book, *The Loneliness of the Long Distance Runner* (1962) is included in my all-time top ten films ever seen. Along with *A Taste of Honey* and *Kes* and many more British classics, this filmic work of art definitively encapsulates working class life in England (Nottingham in this case) in the 1960s. Written by Alan Sillitoe and brought to the screen by Tony Richardson, the film sees Michael Courtney and Michael Redgrave playing characters on opposing sides of the British class divide. The depiction of the realist harshness of life in that era is masterfully crafted for the screen.

As the film opens it sets the criminal substance of what to expect. Michael Courtney's voice narrates, "Running has always been a big thing in our family; especially when running away from the police."

The Loneliness of the Long Distance Runner starts in the present but fluctuates between the present and the past as we, the viewer, start to understand the circumstances that built up to the lead character's current predicament.

Punctuated by gritty quips, the film tells the story of Colin Smith, beset with a mighty chip on his shoulder resenting the class system and his impoverished working-class upbringing, who then turns to petty crime instead. Memorable moments in the film include the rain-soaked scene where Colin gets caught by the police for 'the bakery job' and sentenced to a period of borstal training.

The fact that Colin is discovered to have a talent for cross-country running in borstal is somewhat extraneous to the greater significance of the story which makes political statements via dialogue between the characters. Smith's talent for running though does not just define the ending of the film but projects as a slow moving undercurrent that flows through the narrative.

For effect, the long distance running idea is featured significantly, which sets the scene for the final twist and Smith's final act of defiance against the system he despises.

Out With the Old and
In With the New

The penny dropped a couple of hours after Jeremy Corbyn had won a landslide victory in the Labour Party leadership contest in September 2015, with some 60% of the vote, in that something momentous had happened and the liberal elite were running scared.

This was confirmed when Foreign Secretary Michael Fallon said on BBC News in sinister and threatening tones that the Corbyn result was "A threat to our national security, our economic security and your family's security."

This sort of scaremongering tactic might have worked with the more sensitive and naive amongst us, if the employment minister Priti Patel had not gone on air just after to repeat exactly the same statement, in exactly the same order, on exactly the same news channel verbatim. Big mistake guys; although I must admit it was a good try. Next time try communicating your contrived stories before you televise.

To change the subject slightly but keeping with the same subject matter, although the landslide victory for Corbyn was attained by a massive endorsement from all the Labour groupings, I must say, on *Newsnight* the night before yours truly had an inkling that something had most definitely shifted.

It was what one would call pure drama which will hopefully become more commonplace on the show, a show that in the past has always been determined by a monied figure directing through the presenter's ear-piece. Not this time. It was *Newsnight* host James O'Brien's direct quizzing of the Conservative MP for Shrewsbury and Atcham, Daniel Kawczynski, regarding the Saudi-led coalition air strike in Yemen that killed civilians (even the UN had declared the bombing illegal) which rendered many at home to reel in gleeful surprise.

In fact, Mr Kawczynksi threatened legal action for what he construed as a 'rude, aggressive and patronising' interview.

On another note, the local implications regarding the massive Corbyn mandate are that those who had deserted Labour because the organisation had become another version of the Tory Party (including myself, whose parents and grandparents were keen Labour supporters) can now return. In addition, those who were demonised as 'Militants' and 'Trotskyites' and subsequently frozen out of their traditional movement because they exercised a social conscience can come back to the fold too.

Yes, having voted for Labour myself in the past I am thinking of joining as a paid-up affiliate (if it were not against the rules because I ran as an Independent). I could in fact suggest new ideas and monitor the new Labour Party trajectory in that the party members shall direct policy. Locally, it seems the Labour come Tory council in Newcastle-under-Lyme is in dire need of help. The latest campaign by the council in the summer of 2018, was to waste valuable funds bombarding us with the born in Newcastle-under-Lyme circus owner Philip Astley (who apparently invented the modern circus in 1768). Sorry to burst the bubble of the brain washing campaign folks (Astley propaganda has seen Astley galleries in town, shopping arcades have been named after him, Astley circus visuals can be seen on buses/ billboards, there are circular project inscriptions on pavements and there is even a theatre show all about Philip Astley – talk about in your face), the public of Newcastle-under-Lyme just don't buy it even if the council have Astley's face plastered all over their wheelie bins. To invent the modern circus is not innovative or original; mistreating animals at circuses has been around since the Roman times.

Moreover, the undertaking by the council to widen the pavement on Knutton Lane with a cycle path has gone down like a lead balloon. Few use the cycle lane which I can bear witness to because I walk on it every day. I might have a suspicious mind, but widening the pavement appeared more about shuttling herds of students up to the nearby college than any green initiative. And to think, these public funds could have been used to tackle the disrepair prevalent all over the borough, we could have seen cash incentives to sort out the catastrophic parking problems or even seen monies invested in the councils not fit for purpose complaints process.

Turning back to the idea of joining the Labour Party, I must declare that I did well with my little (but well formed) ninety-four votes when first standing as an Independent in the Newcastle Town ward local elections in 2014, especially as the Lib Dem candidate only polled 125 votes.

Even the Tories admitted my dynamic leaflets were the toast of the campaign.

Perhaps I could be like Anthony Wedgwood Benn (not Hilary, of course, who had initially been named shadow foreign secretary in Corbyn's new cabinet).

I might not have a peerage to renounce but I can write a good piece on the Wedgwood Museum.

Yes, I have decided. I am going to knock on the door of the Labour Party HQ in Newcastle (see image) being as I only live around the corner and ask if there is any room at the inn.

If Paul Farrelly should then enquire as to who I am I could always say, 'Don't you know who I am? I am that unpaid social campaigner who speaks out for ordinary people including the marginalised and the vulnerable – not the privileged few. That principled one who managed to petition to get the potholes in Dunkirk completely resurfaced. I am also the individual (not the party) who lobbied to get the smashed street signs and dangerous bus shelters replaced and am the person who persuaded the relevant authority to transform the scruffy broken down fences in nearby Montgomery Court.'

He will know what I mean.

Who knows, if I do join, perchance MP for Newcastle-under-Lyme, Paul Farrelly and I will be on first name terms. Then we could team up with Mr Farrelly's (sorry Paul's) Labour-Tory-Lite mates Tristram (now defunct) Ruth and Rob (also now defunct) over the border, becoming one big happy family; unity and 'broad church' is the name of the Labour game, you know. Besides policy, compassion in every sense of the word is the political name game too. Never fear, during this difficult time I could always put a reassuring arm around Trist's shoulder and tell him to not be so glum now his prominence has been diminished to that of director of London's Victoria and Albert Museum. After all, he is safe in the knowledge that his book is still flying off the shelves in the Potteries Museum and Art Gallery in Hanley.

Isn't it?

What Species are these Monstrous Creatures?

I will never forget watching the horror-cum-serial killer movie *Seed*. The animal cruelty depicted at the beginning of the picture would make even the toughest recoil in disgust. Priding myself on being pretty hard, I could never watch those images again.

Moreover, the recent furore regarding dogs and cats in China being skinned alive for food and clothing led me to a link which showed raccoons also being skinned alive for their fur. The film is not for the faint-hearted.

It is not macabre to watch such footage; we need to see the horror first-hand so the significance of the brutality can permeate our very being, perhaps to figure out what species these monstrous creatures are (and I don't mean the raccoons). After watching the short clip, I was darkened by both sadness and doubt in relation to what sort of world we live in and how that world corresponds with the notion of an all-powerful God or superior force presiding over it.

It is accepted that here in England we put cows and pigs (and little lambs) through a similar terrifying process the Chinese put cats and dogs through – but the wanton torture as depicted in the video plummets animal cruelty to an unknown baser and more sinister level.

In my view, the chink in the armour of the religious idea that there is a God lies in the animal question. As in how we deem it fine to kill other animals for food and clothing, somehow believing it to be our divine right?

How can we assume moral superiority when we are also animals? Therefore, is the animal torture shown in the video a distortion of this moral superiority human beings hold over other animals? Darwin did prove beyond all doubt that as human beings we are no more than modern apes ourselves and share exactly the same body organs and senses as most other animals, including insects.

It appears that all life on earth is selfish and ruthless when push comes to shove; in that we will kill each other and other animals to survive. But what sort of God would oversee an earth characterised by that premise? In order to reproduce and leave our genes (by our offspring) on this planet, we are instilled with an unexplained and deep-rooted magnetism or conditioning force linked to the procreative act. This is in light of the fact that the earth is not unequivocally and universally appealing to all that dwell on it.

One response is that all animal life derives from the same genus and when we eat a freshly butchered pig, for example, (a bacon or sausage sandwich I think we refer to it as) or a lion kills and eats a zebra, it is ourselves eating ourselves for the sole purpose of life itself surviving, which for some, could take the naked brutality out of the act of killing for food.

But what about the animals that are unfortunate enough to find themselves in the lower echelons of the food chain pecking order, like battery-farmed chickens and rabbits? The latter are terrorised and savaged by those same dogs we mourn over for being killed and eaten by the Chinese.

Then we have the imbeciles in Denmark trying to prove a point by killing and eating a baby rabbit on air. Most of us already understand natural selection in the sense of the hypocrisy regarding the distinction of which animals are deemed a good dinner and which animals are not. After all, a ten-year-old child can recognise that animal flesh is animal flesh.

In addition, there is the beloved pussy cat that is primed to torment the little mouse before executing it. How does that fit into the grand scheme of things on this wonderful dog eat dog planet of ours?

Yes, there are moral and religious dilemmas that can never be explained, but what we do know is that the torture as seen on the video should be stamped out by international agreement with immediate effect and the creatures who perpetrated the barbarism brought to justice.

Furthermore, analytic discourse relating to the moral, religious and even scientific questions regarding our relationship with other animals on the planet needs to be comprehensively ascertained.

Naval Blue

Colours have always perplexed. Why people choose them, wear them, live by them and even die by them. When I visit any town centre I never fail to calculate what colours are predominating by the clothes the general public are wearing at that particular time; and the possible reasons why. This on-the-spot data analysis does not just conclude the obvious hand-me-down explanations, such as wearing white means purity, wearing green could signify the environment and attiring in black could codify bereavement.

Colours also feature largely in art including written text or prose. Dusty rose-pink are just a couple of expressive tasters to illustrate how our 'would be' writers vie to be colour-unique in choosing the right colour phrase for those standardised, overcooked storybook clichés.

Like the darkening of red into burgundy, colour symbolism can appear much deeper. Who marshals the colour schemes in deeming which colour is fashionable and what secondary colours should complement the colour in question (to avoid jarring) is also a curiosity. Colour contrasting patterns, corresponding with different modern eras, emerge today just like they did in Roman times. The difference being that only Caesar could wear a purple toga in the days of the sumptuary laws. If one of the plebeians or even a member of the nobility dared to wear the colour purple they could be put to death.

In England during the mediaeval period, the sumptuary laws were still enforced with regard to what colour apparel one could adorn. It is recorded that in the Elizabethan period, 'puke' (a khaki green colour) 'rat grey' and 'goose turd green' were the in colours only the poorest in society would don. No doubt if yours truly was around in those days, he would have been put to death too, not for breaking the sumptuary laws, but for advocating that the aristocracy wear 'verbal diarrhoea mustard' to contrast their pompously bulbous puffed-up pink faces and blackened forked tongues.

On a different note, we have our modern political parties who govern by the representation of one particular colour or another. Indeed, colour is very important for control in more ways than one. Colour used in modern-day British politics has been reminiscent of a mind-numbing wearisome traffic light, predictably and periodically interchanging from blue, red, and amber and back again.

Let's archive grey-scale politics for another day, I find it simpler and more fun to characterise colour in real lay terms like when I recently visited Portsmouth's Historic Dockyard in Hampshire (October 2017). In the Mary Rose Museum, information regarding the illegality of wearing certain colours in the 16th century is featured, which helped lead to the colour theme associated with this article. Another lead was acknowledged after boarding the boat to Gosport to view the World War 2 naval submarine, *Alliance*. I could not help but notice that the majority of visitors (including myself) had chosen to wear navy blue on that particular day. I had complemented my naval-coloured jacket with air force blue slacks, which could have been keeping in with military (RAF) colour coordination according to those skilled in the subliminal. Therefore, was the naturally inherent seafarer (in us all) pronouncing itself via the psyche by nailing this particular navy blue colour to our own personal masts to make our own personal statements? Furthermore, are we all predisposed to a maritime or marine disposition having more than likely evolved from the seas ourselves? In my colour case (attiring in both naval and air force blue) perhaps I felt my ancestors originally came to being from both the sea and/or the air, or better still, was my chosen colour code suggesting that it was the mammoth modern-day aircraft carrier anchored in Portsmouth docks that I really wanted to board?

What's more, having purchased a multi-ticket (I was not missing out on any of the Dockyard attractions), I wondered why I had asked the tour guide if black was the original colour of the *Alliance*. Was I more than likely thinking nautically, such as water camouflage and the whole spectrum of shades that determine the colours of our seas in which underwater vessels can hide?

Seaing was not relieving though at the Mary Rose Museum after viewing the excellent 1545 Tudor shipwreck recovered from the Solent. Exhibited in the same building were numerous wreckage displays, one of which included the front toothless skulls of crew members (or hands) who had sailed on that fateful day. I did not just imagine the pain the serfs had gone through back then, but also colour imagined the 'grimy green' and 'black gravestone' hues their gnashers must have appeared. Phraseology to one side, I empathised with their tortuous aching which was no doubt compounded by other illnesses/diseases. Prolonged tooth pain is anything but amusing.

Last but not least, colour is so important that it represents what country we herald from (emblems) and throughout the ages no ship that set sail from Portsmouth harbour would have done so without a corresponding colourful ensign. It's worth pondering, therefore, why the *Victory*, in which Admiral Nelson fought the Battle of Trafalgar (1805), was colour coordinated a noteworthy brown and cream.

Thompson Mode
Defining 80s Music

There is some criticism of the 80s music genre today, but it must be said when it was good it was very good and when it was bad it was cringe-worthy. Let's look at the greats. Kraftwerk, a-ha, OMD, Thompson Twins. Thompson Twins? Yes, formed in 1977 and named after two fictional detectives in the now topical *Tintin* series, they disbanded in 1993.

Their greatest hits album does not just feature classics like *Love on Your Side* but the more class acts like *We Are Detective*. Yes, often put on the jukebox when I was a lad, one was usually too intoxicated or preoccupied to understand the full quality. On top of that, one did not have the latest technology of the stereo headphones to appreciate every note, sound, and clever composition that defined the tune like one can today.

We Are Detective begins with a sound appearing so mysterious and covertly effective that it sets the tone for introducing the cloak and dagger concept. This instrumental sound intersperses throughout the track just before the chorus – which brings about the only criticism of the song; the chorus appears laborious.

What distinguishes a great song from an average song is that great songs tell a story. They also have a beginning, a middle and an end. *We Are Detective* delivers on that arrangement.

Staying with the 1980s, it's a difficult question to answer as to what your favourite record of all time is/was. After all, there are so many musical genres and multiples of one's favourite musical tracks. What do some tunes do to us, one could ask, and how do we identify with them?

And why do certain musical compilations inspire, move, galvanise and uplift us?

One song that is most definitely up there for me is *Sea of Sin*, Depeche Mode, 1990 (B-side of *World in My Eyes* single). The single also includes *Happiest Girl* and many versions of *World in My Eyes*.

During my younger days Depeche Mode were personified for some as being a little melancholic, but for others they tendered the allure of robust realism embedded in meaningful lyrics delivered via a new and upbeat electronic sound. Music lovers during the early Depeche Mode years were looking for a message within a song to correspond with the melody. Depeche Mode were definitely geared towards musical connoisseurs who were tired of love-themed lyrics featured in many popular songs of the day. We wanted to hear an insightful story.

To last so long and still produce quality is another major feat for Depeche Mode. We have all borne witness to those making comebacks and making absolute fools of themselves in doing so. In saying that, *Spirit*, released by Depeche Mode in March, 2017, does not do it for me personally.

Sea of Sin opens with an eerie melodic beat that recurs throughout the tune which encapsulates the 'other side of the track' mood. Ironically, this piece could be talking about love but the darker side of it. In addition, the sadness really envelopes the listener when the atmospheric background strain finally plays the song out for the last time; the sadness not being because of the quasi-supernatural nature of *Sea of Sin*, but for the fact the strain did not go on for longer.

The Marl Hole

Vale Place is an area in Stoke-on-Trent Central, a sort of suburb of Hanley that spreads out in a north-westerly direction towards the outskirts of Cobridge. It was named after Port Vale Football Club who used to play at the Old Recreational Ground, Bryan Street, Hanley, until 1950.

My earliest recollections of the locale are around the year 1967. Imprinted on my mind are the event/s when young women used to pick me up and ask me to sing *Puppet on a String* by Sandie Shaw. I always obliged even as a five-year-old and enjoyed the attention even though a little bewildered by all the ado.

Through the eyes of the entranced child, the Vale Place area of Hanley pre-Forest Park was an adventure ground on a mammoth scale featuring gang huts the size of disused factories (Brookfield Foundry) which all radiated that familiar faint metallic, rustic-abandoned smell. There was also rich and varied wildlife to experience around the Hollies (or the 'Ollies as they were vocalised) which was a grass area around the marl hole accessed from an entry at the top of Boundary Street/bottom of Bryan Street. The marl hole was fenced off with black oblong boardings but there was always a way into this man-made industrial-type lake. There was no doubt plenty of flora and fauna around too, but by all accounts I would probably be setting fire to it being as I was a bugger for lighting grass fires. It was especially exciting when the dry, brown, coarse bracken went up in flames thus interspersing with an orange and yellow crunching glow to then disappear forthwith. The black scorched earth aftermath enabled that special burnt smoke smell to cling to the air and to one's clothes for days after.

Large brown satin-coated caterpillars could also be found on those long purple-budded flowers that you now see alongside train tracks. Then we had butterflies such as Frenchies and Cabbage Whites gracefully flitting around. Dragonflies, grasshoppers, tiddlers, darters, newts and the funny-looking baby toads, together with tadpoles and spawn, were also engaged with. The differing stages of metamorphosis from tadpole to toad and the physiological changes that would occur would repeatedly be subject to examination. It was also commonplace to house a pet toad in your back yard; probably in the outside WC.

Specimens could be observed by overturning big duckers (boulders) to see what was underneath. I recall one time, under one stone, amongst the different species of insects seeing a strange-looking creature which I now believe to have been an albino newt/lizard. I distinctly remember that it was white and lightly speckled with black dots. Conversely, if you were also to lift one of those grey pieces of tin sheets with grooves, and you were quick enough, you would see a field mouse run like lightning which was a rare thing to see, believe it or not.

I am not saying we were tough, but we never vacillated when catching bees and wasps in our hands (bees would not usually sting but wasps would). It was the natural order of the day.

As well as the animal characters there were also many human characters interacting with the wildlife, they were called children who lived in the vicinity. There was Jinxie the gang leader who wore glasses (woe betide anyone who dared call him 'Glassy Glitter'). We had Owen, who was short but tough, Bleegan, who was a crack shot, Fur, a fair-headed boy who sometimes spoke through the corner of his mouth, Remus, the easy-going type and brothers John and Anthony Watlins (John being the eldest by one year), who were both often belittled by the others in the group.

I can vividly recall the time when we all stood at the top of the marl hole bank and I spotted a dead Dalmatian dog in the water below. The slimy carcass appeared to be marinating in the stale pool, half-submerged half-floating, in a watery limbo of its own. We knew it was a Dalmatian because of its black and white pelt.

"I can drag that out," John said.

"Go on then, John," I encouraged, "we can build a fire and roast it."

The gang then stood at the top of the marl hole bank to watch John run down and heave the dead canine heavyweight up quite a slope. I can see it now and hear myself commenting as the dappled fur burnt and crackled over a large, well-lit fire; the skin underneath looking white in appearance.

"It looks like bread," I had remarked.

'Doffers' were also commonplace during the Vale Place epoch and one such dare included letting off air bombs (around Bonfire Night) in old abandoned houses to then run around the room attempting to avoid the exploding ball. Talking of old houses, they were another pastime. Not just content with smashing windows, seeing what people had left in their vacated terraced and making a fire in the grate with old furniture to warm up – all while playing pontoon for coppers – was to die for.

Anthony Watlins was more skint than the rest of us and boy, we were skint. He was not only ridiculed, he was bullied, dismissed and always picked last for games. I remember playing pontoon with him across from the Church Wall on Paddock Street, which was adjacent to his humble abode that backed onto the 'Square' where we would play Pitch and Toss. On that occasion he had an unprecedented run of luck and took my money. I kept saying, "Just one more game."

"No, I'm going in now," Anthony said. He then hesitated and glanced at me as if to say that he was up for a few more games but needed coaxing.

"Oh come on."

"Oh, okay then, you deal and give 'em a good shuffle."

Anthony did give me a chance to win my money back but as it turned out it wasn't my day. I was usually gutted when I lost at gambling being as I was one of the best at Pitch and Toss. One Saturday morning, a sizeable crowd had drawn around my house after I had lost my pocket money early on by gambling. The shock of losing my coins so early, thus bringing my day to a premature close (as I saw it), caused me to burst out crying. I was not accustomed to being on the losing side and it was an extremely unwelcome vicissitude. On looking back, it seems almost endearing that a crowd of friends had gathered outside my house to ask my mum if I was okay. They were not there to offer half-arsed banalities, but were genuinely concerned about my wellbeing.

With regard to Anthony, I never did ridicule him myself; it was not in my nature to pick on and expose personal character imperfections.

Anthony's older brother John got just as much stick as Anthony even though he was a strapping lad. He was nicknamed 'Monkey'. John eventually rebelled after being pushed to breaking point and fought with the gang leader Jinxie and surprisingly got the upper hand. We were all shocked and enthralled by John's courage. John was never called Monkey again. In my later years it became known that Anthony had died early in his thirties. I saw him once in the 1990s outside the civic offices in Stoke. On that occasion he appeared to exude mental health difficulties and smoked a lot.

Fascinating Vale Place was also accredited with the Old Mill (another disused factory) assault course on Paddock Street which we negotiated with some agility. It is recalled that on one occasion, a bird (a starling, thrush or blackbird) had rested on top of an oil drum obstacle and had subsequently become stuck in the oily black and brown substance. I will never forget how the bird struggled to release itself from the quagmire and in doing so, immersed itself deeper and deeper into the spillage. Keeping with the bird element but on a happier note, around the Vale Place area one would regularly see flocks of sparrows, a feathery friend which today has all but become extinct.

Best not forget those other childhood games played in this era. There was the 'Pile On' game where everybody piled on top of each other and you had to have a turn being at the bottom of the pile. It was not nice being on the bottom as more often than not it rendered you unable to breathe.

Then there were the interesting amusements associated with the main leisure activity of making fires, initiated as a focal point to which local children assembled. After building such fires it was not always potatoes we would put on. On occasion, small glass bottles full of our own urine would be placed onto the fire as a sort of water bomb, timer and all.

"Let's go over the spare ground and make a fire and see who's about," suggested Fur.

"Shoulds," I retorted. "Yeah, I'm going to whizz in a bottle and put it on."

"Go on then," said Fur.

Fur smirked as I picked up a label-less small glass bottle complete with a lid. I subsequently urinated into it and screwed the top on tight. It did not take long to get a fire drawn. We used wood or flammable debris collected from the spare ground. Mattress stuffing was a good ignitor. Others had gathered at the fire by this time, one being Jinxie. I casually slipped my bottle of urine into the hottest part of the outdoor oven, under some red glowing wood, just as one would do with a potato. Knowing that water bombs would take a while to heat up and 'go off', we would while away the time laughing, joking, telling stories and being children, without the shackles of parental supervision of course.

Suddenly, there was a loud pop accompanied by a *ssssissing* noise. We all laughed out loud

"Fuckeen 'ell that got me," Jinxie, the leader of the gang, gruffed.

This was my cue to run through the nearby entry which led to the bottom of Trafalgar Street where an in-production, cream-coloured pot bank stood. I can still sense the noise the outside grills on the factory walls used to make when discharging the odour of dry clay and dust.

Jinxie caught up with me there and then and that's all he did, catch up with me. We both then walked back to the others surrounding the fire. Perhaps he just had to demonstrate to the rest of the gang that he had done something about the exploding mishap.

Occasionally we were allowed to go camping, which was an excuse to run wild at night. One such night, I recall that a few of us hid in a wooded area by the 'Newty' which was another sort of industrial reservoir, a little smaller than the marl hole, where one caught newts. Then, at about five in the morning, looking yonder towards the Sneyd Street side of the pond, a bright circular light begin to rise slowly.

"Look the sun's cumeen up," I innocently exclaimed.

Jinxie started to laugh out loud, not a titter, but a full body laugh. "It's not the sun yer tit; it's the Rozzers with a search light." At this we all just sat and stared, a little confounded by the beaming light, under cover and obscured by deep dark foliage contrasting a sallow-white pottery slag heap. We were famous.

Why else would we be under the spotlight.

Silly Willie

It seems our Katherine Hepburn soundalike, William Hague, has been at it again – blundering, that is. It all started in March, 2011 for our then incompetent Foreign Secretary, after establishing a no-fly zone over another's country (Libya), Silly Willie could not explain how a Libyan aircraft was shot down.

It does not stop there. 'Initially Willie' could not wait to meddle in Libya and when he got wind of a rebellion the clangers dropped faster than bombs over Tripoli. Even our special forces had been captured because Willie could not wait to 'rush out' and poke his nose in the oil-rich lands to make sure his associates would always be quids in.

His gaffer, David Cameron, backed his Willie though, and played it down because his Tory chum (Willie) could not speak for himself – Willie was busy rushing around to Buckingham Palace to brief the queen that Gaddafi was fleeing to Venezuela. Yes, another gaffe from our Willie.

Last, but not least, never in human history has the British government supported rebel forces. Silly Willie Nilly, though, publicly stated that Britain supports the rebels in Libya. After expelling diplomats from the Libyan embassy in London, Willie was the last to know that the leader of the Libyan rebels, General Abdel Fattah Younes, was shot by his own side.

You're one hell of a Silly Billy; aren't you silly Willie Nilly?

Intermittence or Abstinence

Much is being debated within addiction circles today, not just with regard to the treatment for substance misuse/addiction and how to manage the condition, but the theories behind those who mentor and manage the individuals. This can manifest in different agencies 'sparring it out' due to their respective belief systems.

In one corner we have those advocating controlled using (as in ingesting intoxicants like alcohol and cannabis intermittently) and in the other corner we have the unequivocal voice of total abstinence, period. The obvious conclusion that one can draw is that controlled using can and does lead back to full-blown misuse.

One is never enough for the addict, who, in turn, needs to not just change their habits when in recovery, but to reevaluate their whole way of thinking. Perhaps it is true to say that controlled substance use can keep the addict in the using loop. Even though rewiring is thought to give the addict the best chance of survival, some addiction agencies operate under the remit that heroin addicts can also function in our communities and even become recovery champions themselves if they are being stabilised by controlled doses of the heroin substitute methadone. This almost seems a contradiction in terms. One can understand that controlled using is not as dangerous as fully abusing, but the message given out to those in addiction from those working in addiction (and using a substance) is not as powerful a voice as the voice from those that are for total abstinence.

The argument has also been posed as to the fact that there are those working in the addiction domain who suffer from painful physical conditions and thus are being prescribed opiate-based pain killers to alleviate that pain – should they not become recovery champions? In answer to that dilemma, first of all it would have to be established if that champion/mentor could switch to a non-opiate substitute – we all know the dangers of becoming addicted to opiate-based prescription drugs.

There is also the predicament of whether potential recovery champions should be able to take prescription drugs within the benzodiazepine family like diazepam or valium and still mentor. It can be said that some drugs within the benzodiazepine type are indeed mind-altering and can produce a drowsy state and slurred speech; so should those acting in a professional capacity be under this influence when assisting those trapped in addiction? There are health and safety issues to consider.

Abstinence is the clean way forward and is the knockout blow for controlled usage. Furthermore, abstinence covers those gaps which could enable that destructive demon to creep back in (which can and does occur with controlled usage). Abstinent Recovery Champions (ARC) are also safe in the knowledge that one is best rid of all the intoxicants, to be fully confident and operational when engaging with the difficult and troubled mind of the addict. One lapse for those in recovery can lead to rapid self-destruction and even death.

The Secret Courts

It is thought that Wanda Maddocks was the first person to be imprisoned by the Court of Protection for contempt of court. I would argue that I was, but my jail sentence was suspended.

Since the jailing of Ms Maddocks in a secret court, senior judges have contemplated the prohibition of imprisonment for those in contempt of court unless the hearing is in public. The then Justice Secretary Chris Grayling wrote to the chief judge of family justice to ask him to include the Court of Protection in any such review into the operations concerning the family courts, such was the political fallout surrounding the Maddocks case. Her crime being to remove her own father from a care home believing he was in peril by being resident there.

But what is being missed and still going unreported is the role legal officials from councils had or have in the process surrounding the secret courts.

Apparently, no record of Judge Cardinal's ruling on Ms Maddocks was published and secrecy rules forbade anyone to name the council who had requested that Ms Maddocks be imprisoned. The social worker who gave evidence against her could not be named either.

The veracity of my real-life account below can be verified by a well-known solicitor in Birmingham who represented me at the Priory Courts in Birmingham on July 1st 2011.

I was given a sentence of six weeks' imprisonment, suspended for two years. It was meted out on July 1st 2011, by the same judge who tried Wanda Maddocks and it ran until July 1st 2013.

I had been to previous hearings to try and obtain Court of Protection (like a power of attorney) for my mother who had Alzheimer's disease (the council held Court of Protection at this time) and during one sitting in April 2011, at the Priory Courts in Birmingham, three council representatives (including one from finance) turned up for a ten-minute hearing for one of them to say a short sentence. The local authority's fees eventually stood at £7,338.20 including VAT, coupled with the cost of the committal application at £3,968.45.

I then tried to publicise what had been going on at the courts, such was the injustice regarding the bias shown towards the council, who were determined to hold on to Court of Protection themselves at any cost. Because I dared to attempt to publicise the case I was charged with contempt. I was on no order from a judge and had not breached any injunctions or anything else.

On the 21st June 2011, at approximately 8.45pm, someone was banging on my front door for fifteen minutes and shouting through the letterbox. I was petrified and did not answer. I believed it to be representatives from the legal team at the council because the next day I received an email from their legal department. It said that the council had applied to the Court of Protection to commit me to prison and they wanted to serve me personally to appear at Birmingham Priory Courts on the 1st July 2011.

As such I did not feel comfortable signing anything. When I did appear at the courts on that date, prison officers (or something like Group 4) were patrolling what I now know to be the secret court staring at me as if preparing to take me away. I was a quivering wreck.

I left the court after receiving the suspended jail sentence, feeling degraded, hurt, confused angry and as though I had been abused.

The solicitor who had been nominated by the judge to represent me (I was acting in person) stated in writing that it is against Court of Protection rules to publish anything about the proceedings that had just occurred and I would be sent to prison if I disobeyed.

She said very little at the hearing but did say in person after sentencing that I was extremely lucky because I had dodged two massive bullets. One, because I did not go to prison and the other, because the costs of the hearing had been set against my mother's home.

I did not feel extremely lucky.

Last but Not Least on *Match of the Day*

The BBC complaints department responded with predictable aplomb regarding the screening process on their *Match of the Day* programming of 2012. It was asked of them to explain why, in many cases, Manchester United are listed first on the show and clubs like Stoke City are listed last (it is understood that on many occasions, the brand of football being played at Stoke merited last place).

It was also suggested to the BBC that they conduct historical statistical analysis to ascertain that, if the entertainment stakes were marginal in any given game, how many times have United been favoured to be screened first. Politics in football was also discussed by the complainant, regarding possible bias in the screening process. For example, it was suggested that generic control of the game by United was self-perpetuating by the BBC, in so much as the broadcasting company prefer projecting the United image above that of any other club in the Premier League.

The complainant argued that this reflected the principle that Manchester United had become the richest club over the years by default. In that, historically, the BBC have repeatedly favoured them, which is the reason why United have remained the most powerful club in football. United then cement their dominance in their over-projection by becoming even richer which enables them to buy the best players and be the most entertaining. The cycle of 'the richest rules in football' then continues (or words to that effect).

A representative from the BBC complaints department said in response:

"*Thanks for contacting us regarding Match of the Day broadcast on BBC One. We understand that you were unhappy with coverage on Match of the Day because you felt that Stoke City didn't get enough coverage or credit where it was due and that too much time was spent discussing Manchester United. This issue has been brought to the attention of Paul Armstrong, the editor of Match of the Day and this is a brief outline of his explanation. 'Since regaining the Premier League highlight rights in August 2004, our aim has been to provide a more comprehensive review of Saturday's Premier League action. It's our intention that we do not show less than five minutes of a game – in fact we frequently show more. The running order for each programme is determined by the day's big stories, talking points and most entertaining games. There is certainly no perceived bias against or in favour of certain teams. Each match takes its place in the running order on its own merit. And it is precisely for that reason that we send a commentator to every Premier League game on Saturdays and Sundays. Nevertheless, we'd like to assure you that your feedback has been registered on our audience log. This is a daily report of audience feedback that's made available to many BBC staff, including members of the BBC Executive Board, programme makers, channel controllers and other senior managers. The audience logs are seen as important documents that can help shape decisions about future programming and content.'*

Thanks again for taking the time to contact us."

Indirect Manslaughter Commonplace in Care Homes

First of all, let me say that it has been consistently vocalised that I did not want my mother moved from the care home where she had been resident for some five years because she was at end of life, extremely ill/fragile with progressed Alzheimer's disease and she was eighty-two. I thought the move would kill her and said so on BBC Radio just after the care home announced I had four weeks to find her alternative accommodation because it was closing down.

After wrangling with a potential new care home as to whether they would take my mum or not, they did so after I contacted a senior manager. My mother arrived at that new care home on the 21st of December 2016. Subsequently, she ate hardly anything for the next twelve days and appeared very ill even though at her previous care home it had been reported that she was eating well. Then on December 31st 2016 (twelve days after the move) I received a telephone call from the deputy manager of the new care home who said my mum was bleeding from down below.

I stated that I did not want my mother to go to hospital because of her fragility. In addition to that, I had already agreed that because my mum was on end of life care she would not be taken to hospital but nursed in the home if she became ill, taking into consideration the distress it would cause her to be processed through the hospital system. She was a vulnerable adult. The care home staff member said there was no paperwork regarding palliative care for my mother so she had no alternative but to telephone for an ambulance. The ambulance took three hours to arrive. I relayed over the telephone to both the staff member and the paramedic that I was not happy about this situation believing that the ambulance journey would have a detrimental effect on my mother's health, coupled with the fact it was New Year's Eve and Accident and Emergency would be at breaking point.

I then received a telephone call from a consultant at the CDU facility of Accident and Emergency and agreed to convene at the hospital to discuss how to proceed with my mother's care. At the hospital I was informed that my mother had only hours to live and they would make her as comfortable as possible at the CDU facility where she would stay.

The very next day (January 1st 2017) a different consultant advised that my mum could last hours, days or even a week and they were looking at moving her back to the new care home, together with the appropriate palliative care documentation so the home knew how to care for her. He said that my mum's GP should have provided the palliative care plan document even though my mum was in the process of being registered at a new surgery. The mystery of where the palliative care documents were when my mother was resident at her previous care home (if there were any) and why these documents were not passed on to the new care home still needs to be unravelled.

I told the second consultant that to move my mother back to her new care home or to a busy ward there at the hospital was a cruel thing to do in light of my mum's extremely fragile state. The consultant maintained that they had not expected my mum to last this long and I got the impression the bed was needed, as ill patients were lining both sides of two corridors. A & E at this point was an utter chaotic disgrace.

I said I was not happy with the situation and the consultant then informed me that the palliative care team would assess my mum and they would let me know the outcome in due course. The palliative care team telephoned me the same day to say my mum had hours to live and they recommended she should not be moved but she should stay in room 9 on the CDU facility.

My mother then died in the early hours of January 3rd 2017.

The only logical and informed conclusion I can come to, therefore, after thirteen years of problems and battles regarding my mother's poor social health care, is that there are malign individuals hiding behind our institutions who are making decisions which are directly impacting on our health and social care services which, in turn, is allowing sinister scenarios like this one described to be commonplace. This is an abhorrence and has no place in a civilised society. There are also countless institutions, associations, groups and individuals who are complicit in the malevolence. I also believe that actions and decisions taken both by government and the care home system accelerated my mother's untimely death which in itself has criminal overtones. My mother was not ready to die but was, in a fashion, killed off by the forced fourteen to fifteen mile move from her care home. I would claim that my mother had been taken away unnecessarily and aggressively before the natural course of her life was meant to end, which in itself violates the sanctity of life.

Subsequently, the coroner refused an inquest and put my mother's death down to natural causes. As you have just read, there was nothing natural about the events that led up to her death. It can be said that the coroner is the chief cog in the institutional wheel. When I have questioned those institutions involved in my mother's care, in that her death was accelerated by the move and she did not die of natural causes, they quote the coroner's findings to avoid culpability. I was informed by the coroner's office that my mother was one of twenty-three deceased persons waiting in the mortuary for a post-mortem. It was relayed that staff members had convened a meeting to discuss the crisis. For my mother to be forced to wait on some macabre production line to ascertain the cause of her death breaches both the dignity of the deceased and the dignity of the family. According to NHS Guidelines post-mortems are usually undertaken within twenty-four hours or, at the most, three days; my mother's post-mortem took two weeks to organise.

It's a Bus Station:
Not the Second Coming

Never in my life had I heard such a commotion concerning... yes, wait for it... a new bus station. The opening of Hanley bus station in March, 2013, was reported by the local media similarly to what the Russians would do when launching a space rocket.

Working public bus stations (transport) are classed as one of the basic needs that comprise human life, together with food and shelter.

So where does that leave the hunter-gatherers of Stoke-on-Trent?

All the furore regarding the new bus station reinforces the notion to the outside world of what a backward city Stoke-on-Trent is. It's no wonder some 'academics' from outside the area believe it's all well and good to tell 'Stoke Jokes' (on occasion in front of Stoke-on-Trent folk might I add).

Headlines and statements peddled from the local media, like: '*A bus station to be proud of*', '*sends out a positive message about regeneration, investment and confidence in the area*', and a '*driving force in the city's recovery*' is near on embarrassing.

The most humorous utterance regarding all the tomfoolery must go to a First Bus driver obviously briefed as to what to say:

"*It's a true honour to be driving the first bus out of this station,*" he quipped.

The city council leader then got in on the act to voice:

"*For years, people have raised concerns about the state of the old bus station. We have listened to them and worked hard to bring about a new bus station with a breath-taking design.*"

Breath-taking design? Those of us who step outside of the area know full well that these orthodox transport contraptions are dotted all around the country.

The Gladstone Pottery Museum: a Compelling Drama

It seems to be an uphill struggle to watch anything decent on TV these days. Recently, I have had to resort to watching reruns of the original *Upstairs Downstairs* where at least the viewer is guaranteed a half-decent script.

Set in Edwardian London, the dialogue in the hit 1970s series can be thought-provoking too. Phraseology like 'shipshape and Bristol fashion' (meaning come on, get moving, or, it's in good order) and 'cat lick' (meaning not having a thorough wash) was used when I was young. As was 'and lather that face' (meaning use soap instead of just splashing on a drop of water). If one did not use soap one could be goaded with the expression, 'You've got a rim around your neck.'

The most interesting character award in *Upstairs Downstairs* has to go to the mulish and supercilious Nanny Webster. What a laugh she was.

Then we had that other 70s drama, *Clayhanger*, which saw some scenes shot at the Gladstone Pottery Museum. Like the ripple effect, *Clayhanger* then motivates one to wonder as to why a series or even a feature film set in Victorian/Edwardian England cannot be filmed in the Potteries, considering authentic cinematic locations are showcased all around the Gladstone Museum.

A visit to the Gladstone is a humbling experience which enamours the local visitor with a sense of pride, in that the professional skills needed to display such an imaginative historical overview of our industrial heritage would be difficult to emulate even with unlimited finance.

Costing £7.50 (with concessions) and £22 for a family ticket (2017) the Museum on Uttoxeter Road, Longton must be put on your things to see before you die list.

Yes, it's that good.

One can also purchase an annual pass (concessions £9.25) which entitles the visitor to free entry for twelve months. The Gladstone is a nice place to be, whether to have lunch (which is reasonably priced) or for just spending an hour or two.

In parallel to the mechanisms that make for a good film, the Gladstone Pottery Museum also engages, educates and entertains (the triple E rating). One of my personal favourite elements presented at the factory museum is the pottery worker mannequin. Complete with saggar on head inner kiln – which is itself encased in the hovel (the bottle oven) – this particular demonstration proves an innovative hit. In the 18th, 19th and 20th centuries the fierce heat from the kilns was thought to be so unbearable it was a hellish existence for the saggar stackers.

Then we have display number 24, 'Flushed with Pride', which depicts ceramic bathroom fittings. While browsing the rooms, I was most impressed with past representations of the pottery industry (the ethereal Pig and Muck visual included).

An unusual surprise also awaits the visitor in lieu.

Last but not least, the evocative display number 21, The 'Doctor's House', which presents a Victorian doctor's surgery, is a viewing must. In the surgery itself, we learn about the many diseases local people were suffering from during this period (life expectancy was thirty-seven for the pottery workers in the mid to late 19th century). Potter's rot (silicosis) was interminably prevalent at this time where one symptom of the disease was coughing blood. Other common diseases were diphtheria, cholera and scarlet fever.

Even the accents of the recorded local people describing their ails to the doctor are authentic. I could actually envisage actors and actresses billing about the rooms costumed up, acting the part; ready for the next take.

It must be said that in real life there is a paucity of English period dramas featuring the lower classes (except perhaps the Catherine Cookson adaptations).

It is almost as if lower-class lives do not bear any interest because of their standing. Are they not worthy of dramatising? Motifs denoting indignity and abject poverty enmeshed in the God-fearing Victorian/Edwardian social tragedy are well received.

Potteries-themed scripts would make compelling viewing and should come to life again. One can categorically declare that North Staffordshire is ripe for a gritty production demonstrating the archetypal industrial callousness of the time. Yes, there would be room for pompous upper-and middle-class characters like Nanny Webster, too.

With the age of digital remastering, we could see more of our unforgiving, smoke billowing landscape of the day, simultaneously focusing in on real storylines regarding real people.

Longton people, that is.

Getting It in the Neck

You do not have to be young and fit to experience paintballing, but it helps. Costing only around £20 per person (there is a fee for extra cartridges) many would conclude that it is a bargain day out. Usually set in picturesque locations, the paintball site can also be accessed by those who are a little bit older or those with mobility issues too.

When the paintball game commences, waddle over, pick your spot behind a large tree, camouflage yourself with twigs from the forest floor, and just hide there as a sniper. I can tell you that once you do get 'shot' you will not put your neck on the line quite as haphazardly the second time around. My first visit saw a 'baptism of fire' when I got it in the back of the neck. Even the staff at the site felt pity and exclaimed it was the most painful place to be hit. I can just image the excitement displayed by the spiteful long-term visitor who had shot me; they must have thought it was their paintballing birthday when my ripe 'young' neck was exposed and there for the taking. It must be a place the hardened paintballers dream of hitting. Sort of a paintballers bullseye. The rotter.

Don't let that put you off trying paintballing out. It does not hurt enough to deter you from engaging in the battle again; it is a timely reminder that you need to be on your toes. Keeping in mind that, if being a sniper is not your thing, you can always spend the duration hiding behind obstacles like a mound of tyres and 'not come out' for the battle. The sound of paintball shots would deter the bravest amongst us from venturing out in any case. Then if the opposition does come up behind you, you can always pitifully squeal 'surrender' and if you are on the wrong side of forty and/or disabled they might 'let you off'.

Paintballing is a fantastic experience and if a participant does not fancy entering the battlefield period, they can always give strategic advice from the sidelines. One such advice is to explain regarding the seasoned players who specialise in how and where to hit the novices. Then you might not be accessible to getting it in the back of the neck quite so easily.

Pointing the Finger

It went from bad to worse for the Secretary of State for Work and Pensions, Iain Duncan Smith. In 2015, the United Nations were considering investigating the UK government over their welfare reforms to assess whether they have caused 'grave or systematic violations' to the human rights of the disabled.

Having the courage of my convictions back in April of the same year to pose the idea that there was a correlation between those losing their benefits and suicide, I was decried for doing so. Judging by some comments in reference to the article I had written on the subject, it was as if I had stated something monstrous.

Why would anybody castigate someone for raising such an important issue in the public domain? What's more, who are these people? What have they got to gain? What nasty bitterness motivates them and what sort of ugly mutation hides behind the user name?

It then emerged that towards the end of August 2015, 2,500 vulnerable people had died just weeks after being declared fit for work.

In that same article I posited the idea that parallels can be drawn between the subtle persecution of the unwaged to that of being Jewish in 1930s Berlin, for which one commenter berated me for insulting the millions of Jews that had perished under the Nazi regime.

This was in light of the fact that former Job Centre advisor Angela Neville had already told the *Guardian* newspaper that she got brownie points for cruelty and her work almost became the persecution of vulnerable people.

Also discussed in the piece above-mentioned was the theory that the bureaucracies that govern us are helping to push people over the edge. Furthermore, I stated words to the effect that those who escape the anxieties and stresses of repeated form filling by imbibing copious amounts of drugs and alcohol can die as a result, so the real suicide statistics are much higher.

Hypocrisy and ignorance is not just the prerogative of some of the commenters.

We had Labour Party leader hopeful, Andy Burnham, getting in on the act with punitive talk. Having been part of a Labour government that started the persecution ball rolling by introducing the WCA (Work Capability Assessment) and then abstaining on the Tory Welfare Bill, he then declared that the Conservative government is punishing and dehumanising vulnerable people (those in receipt of benefits).

This socio-political tragedy has almost turned into a dark pantomime.

According to Disability Rights UK, DWP call centre workers in Glasgow have been issued with six-point suicide risk guidance for those claimants threatening to take their own lives because of issues with welfare payments. This includes waving a pink laminated guidance notice above their heads if they suspect a caller is suicidal so a manager can rush over to 'gather information'.

There are other institutions as well as the DWP that are bringing unnecessary suffering to the disabled. Take council tax departments for example.

I paid my council tax bill on the 28th July, 2015, for that month but that was apparently too late. On the 21st of that same month, a pink council tax reminder letter had already gone through the system and had been sent out to arrive at the beginning of August 2015. When I questioned this anomaly the council informed me I must pay the tax at the beginning of every month and that people (including vulnerable adults) who don't are only given a certain amount of pink reminders (three or four) before they are summoned to appear before a court like common criminals and threatened with imprisonment.

Talk about the old saying, 'pay or be taken away'.

I then challenged the council to advise what remit they operate this policy under and to provide legal clauses to support the rule that monthly council tax payments must be paid on or around the 1st of the month. The rationale being that it is difficult for those on low incomes to juggle their finances with many having to borrow from Peter to pay Paul. Nowadays there are many more bills to pay and less money around to pay them with.

We all well know that debt has to be paid, but in saying that, local government needs to cut people some slack.

In response to raising the issue, the council sent out reams of dense legal theoretical text to prove their first of the month point, which the majority of the population would find difficult to understand. In turn, such bureaucracy would trigger anxiety and distress even in those who are not disabled or have ongoing mental health problems.

I also asked the council if they are aware that their threatening letters could be contributing to suicide rates locally, in light of the fact that debt is one of the main reasons people take their own life. On top of that, I asked what guidance or help they have in place for those at risk of suicide (like that of the DWP in Glasgow and their pink laminate).

Although still awaiting a response, if I am feeling stressed I could always visit the council tax department in Newcastle waving the perilous pink reminder letter above my head, then perhaps a manager might rush over. I won't be holding my breath though.

No doubt they will make contact 'in due course' (another condescending institutional phrase).

The Corbyn Show

The final Labour Party leader debate in 2015, before the crucial September 12th vote on electing the next Labour leader, and perhaps the new Prime Minister, was aired on Sky News on the Thursday before, with many claiming that quintessentially, the debate manifested as the 'Jeremy Corbyn Show'.

Even pre-event, 66.5% of Sky Pulse users believed that Jeremy Corbyn would poll more favourably. Equally, post-event, 80.7% of those polled believed Corbyn had won the final hustings. Liz Kendall was way behind in second place with 8.5%, Yvette Cooper on 6.1% and Andy Burnham polling just 4.7%.

The same statistics were reflected on social media, where both Twitter and Facebook reported massive support for Corbyn.

In reference to Andy Burnham, during the debate he stuck to his chosen tactic throughout of both straddling the left and right fence simultaneously, which some would say cost him dearly. Neither here nor there, he lacked political mettle, insomuch as he is a likeable guy and that's it I'm afraid, a likeable guy but prime minister material – no.

Liz Kendall, on the other hand, had noticeably changed tack. Doing her best to rinse away that hint of Tory blue, it sort of worked in her strange Dolly Daydream way. We still had the same old drawbridge metaphor coupled with her uniform 'reaching out to the whole country' notion, but to put it bluntly; she is not a convincing orator and takes a little long to deliver the point.

As for Yvette Cooper, together with both Burnham and Kendall, at every opportunity she took a pop at the Conservatives and David Cameron, which was not what the event was about. They just can't help themselves, can they? Cooper displayed most of what the electorate are turned off by in politics (petty bickering and spin).

At one point in the show, the Sky presenter Adam Boulton proceeded to back Cooper, thus posing a ridiculous question to Corbyn on the lines of what the '*Sun* says'. Replying that he did not read the newspaper (or, some would argue, comic, bearing in mind Bunty Brooks is back at the helm) the Islington North MP brought about some loud chuckles from the audience, one of whom reminded Boulton that his personal interrogation of Corbyn was not appropriate (or words to that effect).

After Cooper had finished her now predictable tirade regarding printing money willy-nilly linked to national debt and the economy, she came across well, a little hoity-toity with plenty of 'robusts' (the political in word) thrown in for good measure.

Schoolmarmish Cooper gambled on tackling Corbyn head on and lost.

In all fairness Cooper does have her good points and is very strong on figures. Regarding the current migrant chaos she has suggested that if each town council in England agreed to house ten migrant families we could take in 10,000 people in one month. In saying that, Yvette Cooper is herself adept at 'flipping' her homes, having already done it three times. Perhaps she could flip one over to a refugee family and offer them free board and lodging. After all, she could always claim it back from parliamentary expenses.

In May 2007, both she and Ed Balls moved to a larger £655,000 property in North London which they designated their second home. They also put the bill for the £2000 cost of the removal vans on to their expenses list as well as regularly submitting claims of £600 per month just for food. Yes, they could teach the refugees a thing or two.

Not satisfied with salaries of £141,866 apiece and personal expenses perks to boot, in 2010, Balls and Cooper were referred to the parliamentary sleaze watchdog after claiming more than £14,000 in travel expenses for their children.

Yes, one can safely say that our Yvette is good at sums; sums of money for herself, that is.

Moving on to Jeremy Corbyn and keeping with the refugee topic, I must say I agree with the majority of his policies, but when hearing Corbyn's London-centric deluded opinions on immigration I feel like putting my hands to my ears. Yes, it's a disgraceful set of events with those from Syria, Afghanistan and Iraq desperately attempting to enter Europe and we need to do all we can to help. But there has to be a political solution to the problems in their respective countries to avoid this mass exodus from occurring in the first place.

This might be difficult for some people to understand, in light of the tragic image of a wasted young life washed up on a beach. But the truth of the matter is that many do not want any more immigrants, migrants, refugees, asylum seekers or any other foreign nationals entering Britain, full stop. After examining their consciences, evidence on the ground shows that ordinary British people feel they already have their immigration quotient and would resent a further influx.

To summarise both this article and the Labour leader debate, let's concentrate on some of Mr Corbyn's many pluses and the reasons why he was eventually elected Labour Party leader.

Primarily, he makes perfect sense when espousing a complete rethink on our drugs policy and to bring energy and rail companies back into public ownership. In addition, he has a clear strategy regarding Labour Party activists/members being the ones dictating future Labour Party policy. We also need an end to the disingenuous practice of the parachuting in of those hand-picked to represent safe Labour seats. Local party members should be the ones representing local people at Westminster.

The Hoi Polloi are sick to the back teeth of political representatives sitting on multiple committees and claiming expenses for doing so. How many well-paid jobs can a career politician have at one time one might ask?

Jeremy Corbyn is just the fillip for those who desire the politically refreshing. Although ganged up on through the debate, he still showed great temperance which most definitely points to prime ministerial.

The House on Greenbank Road

Child sexual abuse is a heinous violation of the innocent. So why has it always been so prevalent in British society? We have had historical celebrity/clerical abusers who, because of their supposed status, got away with it for years; we have cases where establishment figures have sexually abused children; and then we have child abuse happening within close family circles (which can include family friends).

There are also cases where older children can pursue the abuser to engage in sexual activity with them. Should leniency against the accused be shown in this instance? One thinks not, as responsible adults we should abide by an unwritten moral code.

In essence, the crime of viewing sexual imagery of children on the internet should warrant a much more serious punishment than community service.

They say that there is no greater love than a mother for her child. Nonetheless, in some instances the mother could have an inkling her child is being sexually, physically or psychologically abused (or all three) but is afraid to rock the boat because the perpetrator of the abuse (their partner) matters more.

The theory that there is no greater love than a mother for her child is therefore defective.

Then we have emotionally mature fifteen-year-old girls who could be engaged in a sexual relationship with an emotionally immature eighteen-year old man; is this sexual abuse or should discretion be used in this scenario?

Child abuse destroys the life of the victim and can lead to drug addiction, mental health problems (including self-harm) and suicide in adult life. Are paedophiles born that way and if they are how can we collectively manage them and initiate an effective deterrent to protect vulnerable children?

Castration is not always the answer, you know.

Having said that, some children are lucky in that memories of their childhood are positive, not negative and disturbing.

I was one such lucky child.

My childhood memories are not of fear and distress but of a belonging security, especially when visiting my grandparents' house on Greenbank Road, Tunstall in the years 1966–69.

Unbeknownst to me, my dad would sometimes sneakily stick his thumb out and hitch it from Hanley to the bottom of Scotia Road in Tunstall. I innocently supposed that it was someone he knew who had stopped to pick us up. One could safely hitch a lift in those days.

We would then cut through that path and over the playing fields onto Greenbank Road via Queen's Avenue. Oddly enough, the goal posts on the green still look the same today as they did all those years ago.

Etched in my long-term memory, even though I was a very young child, is my grandfather's shock of white hair and smiling face when he once came down to greet us at the gate. There are also fond memories of my grandmother reaching for her handbag, as I knew she was about to give me a tanner (sixpence) or even a shilling if I was very lucky.

This would then allow me to visit the outdoor (the shop part) of the Ancient Briton public house (known as the Brit, now demolished) which was just around the corner. En route I would sometimes see the Sunday morning football team changing for the match in a sort of alley on the left-hand side of the pub.

Looking back, one recognises that children have a naive perception of reality. This can be illustrated by the occasion when my aunty, who still lived at my grandparents' house, played the latest Frank Sinatra hit *My Way* on repeat. Nobody even laughed when I seriously remarked that the record should not be continually replayed because Frank Sinatra's voice would become tired.

Cousins could be at the house on Greenbank Road, being as my dad was one of nine. If they weren't, I would either walk over and visit another aunty off Sunnyside Avenue in Mill Hill or stay put and catch bees and wasps in a jam jar.

Fresh vegetables complementing a nice Sunday dinner can also be recalled; Sunday dinners still being my favourite meal today.

Always armed with a pack of playing cards, it was an adventure of the most monumental kind on Greenbank Road. Especially after the Brit had closed for the afternoon and my uncles came back to the house and handed out the dosh. Asking anyone to play a hand with me for money, my dad's brothers even gave me the lucre back if I lost (I do recall a not so nice uncle on my mum's side who I played snooker with for money and lost. And just like Chicken Licken, I thought the sky had fallen in when he kept the money – even though I would have done exactly the same).

The fondest memories of all, though, were experienced when returning home via the bus caught from the stop outside Dudson Ltd on Scotia Road. Confident, safe and content with my newly accrued coppers jingling in my short trouser pockets; I could have taken on the world and won.

Major Flaws in the Government's Alcohol Strategy

The coalition government sang from the same hymn sheet when they formulated their Alcohol Strategy presented to Parliament in 2012. The long-awaited document showed little understanding of the physical and emotional illnesses attributed to mind-altering legal substances like alcohol and the fall-out associated with that dysfunction.

Addiction (including alcohol use), as we all know, is usually compatible with homelessness, offending, domestic violence, sexual impropriety and mental health problems. Then there is the untold social complications and cost to the NHS and our economy.

It has to be said that in the mainstream, understanding of what addiction actually is can be non-existent.

The report does not offer any theories or understanding around the self-destructive nature of alcohol and does not address the pertinent questions. One such concern is that some in our communities who have substance misuse problems and seek help from their doctor could be inadvertently receiving a black mark against their name should a future employer wish to peruse their medical records.

This could deter those with drug and alcohol problems from seeking expert help.

The general consensus is that the paper was published only to appease the alcohol industry and does not offer any solution to the growing socioeconomic problems caused by alcohol carousing other than to contain it by robust over-policing when necessary.

This means that the burden of the problem seems to have been passed on to our local overstretched and underfunded health/social care agencies (including the police) to manage.

The police are not just managing the stereotypical down-and-out nuisance type of alcoholic. They have to contain order in towns throughout Britain where weekend 'benders' enable sections of our society (sometimes high on a cocktail of substances) to descend into a madness which can include mass brawls and widespread social anarchy.

Most people with addiction problems don't do moderation and those on the periphery of full-blown addiction (as in those not classed as having addiction problems but becoming troubled by excessive drinking) must run into the tens of thousands.

The government's manipulation of statistics is also cause for criticism, as in statistical figures seemed to have been pulled out of a hat to suit the argument. For Prime Minister David Cameron (in the PM foreword of the document) to declare that the root cause of our violent binge drinking culture was down to the cheap price of alcohol is thought ludicrous by many currently working in the addiction sphere.

The blueprint also offered no theories behind the causality of binge drinking (such as environmental, social, economic or cultural factors) or problems that could arise by raising the price of alcohol, which could see more of the family income being spent on the drug instead of their dependents.

The most startling persiflage contained in the document can be seen in the introduction, where it is stated that in moderation, alcohol consumption can have a positive impact on wellbeing and can encourage sociability.

It is thought that this false self-confidence (or sociability) supposedly gained from imbibing alcohol should not be encouraged; the reasons being that social drinking could mutate into full-blown alcoholism. This could be seen with the diffident individual eventually becoming reliant on alcohol just to mingle which could see them unable to socialise at all without that prop.

To also say that, in moderation, alcohol can have a positive impact is dangerously misleading. Nothing can compare or impact as positively as the strength of the sober mind in comparison to that of a mind befuddled by alcohol, even in small quantities.

Furthermore, most parents would want their teenage children to integrate with their peers and evolve into adulthood without the need for personality-changing enhancers. Young people should not feel the need to be under the influence of a drug whatever the dosage.

The government's proposals on licensing laws and alcohol distribution also fell under critical spotlight. Curbing alcohol abuse by controlling dispensing times for problematic venues is negated on the basis of the readily available 24-hour supermarkets and the 'Dial a Beer' facility.

In conclusion, restricting the glamorous advertising of alcohol is not included in any future government strategy. There is also no hint of introducing legislation to enable the multibillion-pound drinks industry to contribute to the rising medical/social cost of treating those suffering from long-term alcohol-related diseases.

The Biggest Monkeys of All

It is with a great source of amusement that academics past and present believe that somehow man, the big ape, is different from the rest of the animal kingdom. Take the monkeys in nature reserves, for example; it gets a little tedious examining them when all our closest ancestors seem do all day is eat, defecate, engage in social grooming and run up and down (trees in their case) squawking. Remind you of anybody you might know?

Well, humans spend most of their time preoccupied with gorging anything they can get their hands on too, don't they? Take Nigella Lawson, for instance, on her upmarket cookery show.

Yummy!

She and others like her peddle the myth that it's almost upper-class to butcher another animal and then dress a piece of its flesh up to call it Beer-Braised Pork Knuckles with Caraway and Garlic (or something else as pompously ludicrous). Notwithstanding, Nige's cooking utensils must cost a small fortune.

Yes, Caraway and Garlic detracts from the fact that we are base flesh eaters just like the rest of the carnivores. What's more, Nigella seems to delight in rolling the animal innards out with her hands, filling the giblets with some fancy herb or other. It's propagated as being sophisticated.

It can be argued that animal flesh eating has developed into a self-centred sort of highbrow culinary art, not a necessity. On the menu and titled by ridiculous descriptors such as haute-cuisine or gourmet, are frogs' legs, snails and the boiled-alive lobster. When you break it down, flesh eating is anything but refined.

Yes, us, the big ape; the biggest monkey of them all?

The Paper Cart

Life as a teenager growing up in Rhyl was not just about the amusement arcades, the fair and holidaymakers. The café setting on the High Street played a large part in the social exchanges of the time, as did Woolworths – or 'Woolies' – and the Astra Cinema, now a bingo hall to the right-hand side as you come out of the railway station, nestled beside Vale Road Bridge. The Plaza Cinema on the junction of High Street and Sussex Street, which is now the Piazza restaurant (2018) was also central to all things happening in Rhyl in the years 1975–79.

Café-wise, there was that blue café with the long side window opposite the Plaza, which used to feature a jukebox at the back. Then there was a little Tiko's-like café opposite that, just below the Plaza. Flamingos, on the bus station (both demolished) where we would order pasty and chips can also be called to mind. The bus station was the meeting place – usually at 6pm on weekdays.

Regarding Woolies (now B&M Bargains Store), the record section at the back was always frequented. It was not unusual to stick the latest singles under one's jacket either. I personally remember tea-leafing *Rivers of Babylon*, Boney M, *Boogie Oogie Oogie*, A Taste of Honey and *Use Ta Be My Girl*, the O'Jays. I would also ask a member of staff to play *Work all Day*, Barry Biggs and *Stumblin' In*, sung by Chris Norman and Suzi Quatro.

Outside the Plaza used to stand the paper cart, which was a bicycle with a square box stand at its front where people used to buy a paper and leave their money in the box to pay for it. Of course, we used to raid the paper cart every chance we got. I can still recall the look of disgust the paper cart owner gave me one night – he knew it was us.

I regret raiding the paper cart.

On a more positive note, the Plaza Cinema was also the place to be. I first saw *Jaws* there, but the most exciting was trying to get in to see the X films (over 18). There was Blondie, as we used to call her, who manned the kiosk and sold the cinema tickets. She was an attractive blonde who we chatted to; she allowed us in to see the X films. In contrast, we had Black Betty, as she was aptly named; she was older and had a coarse dyed black mop. There was not a cat in hell's chance she would let us in.

One school friend came up with the novel idea of me wearing a girlfriend's long navy-blue coat, supposedly because it made me look older, before attempting to gain entrance to see an X film. It seemed to work when Blondie was 'on' and getting in outweighed any possible embarrassment factor.

Down at the Astra Cinema, we did not even try to pass for eighteen – because there was no chance. But this did not stop us seeing the X films. We would either sneak in through the exit doors or pay into Astra 2, to see an A (over 12) or an AA (over 14) film, and then sneak next door to Astra 3 to watch the rude X films. It was very exciting sitting there not knowing if we were going to get caught or not.

In 1975, one film I stayed and watched in Astra 2 was *The Towering Inferno*. When the secretary dived out of the tower on fire (now cut) I was most shocked. Not at the actual footage, but because it was the first time I had realised the narrative does not necessarily have to feature happy-endings.

If you are ever on Rhyl High Street walking past the old Plaza, try to imagine a real life stage, not a choreographed one. In this particular clip, enacted some 40 years ago, a group of effervescent young friends of fourteen or fifteen with their whole lives ahead of them would feature. They would be talking excitedly about plotting to get into the flicks to see an X film. One male teenager, may I add, would be attired in a girl's three-quarter length coat.

Greek Bailout 3:
The Director's Cut

There had been a brand new factual filmic blockbuster running on our TV screens in the summer of 2015. Shown live on BBC, Sky and RT News, it was called: *Greek Bailout 3*.

And wasn't it compulsive viewing? The protagonist featured in the starring role (Alexis Tsipras from the governing Syriza Party) swiftly turned into his own antithesis as he dramatically sold out the Greek people with European Union (EU) dictated austerity measures hastily pushed through parliament. This came directly after Syriza had called a referendum in which that same Greek populace overwhelmingly voted against that same austerity.

The contradiction and confusing rationale being that the Greek people want to remain in the EU and the eurozone but at the same time don't want the reforms that come with remaining. One can safely argue therefore that the EU and the eurozone have failed. How come there are supposedly no euros in Greek banks but trillions of euros in German banks when all member states are supposed to be involved in one European single currency? Aren't Germany's euros Greece's euros and vice versa? Why not call a final referendum once and for all as to whether Greece should leave the EU/ eurozone in light of the bail-out terms and subsequent loss of sovereignty? Like many European nations believe, it is common sense for Europe to cooperate as a trading entity. In making this statement though, it must be kept in mind that the monetary dominance of such institutions by some member states, or should I say directors, (Germany in this case), should be legislated against.

On another note, it is not just best practice for European countries to have trade agreements with their continental counterparts, it would also be good practice to have a standard European Health Service free at the point of access.

Turning back to Greece, running parallel to the protagonist in this fascinating Greek drama was the German antagonist Angela Merkel. Yet, her bit-part cronies were also desperate to get in on the act. We saw the arrogant and obnoxious Finnish Prime Minister, Juha Sipilä (my mum would have called him a funny-looking bugger), the Latvian Prime Minister, Laimdota Straujuma, and the Ukrainian Prime Minister, (Ukraine is not even in the EU) Yatsenyuk all get their ten penneth in. How did the above manage to become centre stage in this EU debacle, one wonders? Some would argue that those nations are not even geographically placed to be classed as European. Yes, those who pontificate regarding austerity but do not lead austere lives themselves threw fuel on the fire of protestations outside the Greek parliament as Athens – the birthplace of democracy – smouldered. No good nail-biter, of course, is ever quite complete without good old-fashioned coinage (euros in this instance) featuring; and there seemed to be 'billions of it' but not for them as far as the Greeks were concerned.

Greece being cast as the pauper amongst kings in that failed group of nations called the EU, had nothing it could call its own but the burden of heavy debt. Then dramatically, we all held our breath as the International Monetary Fund (IMF) made their on-screen entrance to state that Greece's debt was 'highly unsustainable'. This was in light of the fact that Greece had already sold its soul (public assets which include land) to its creditors.

It can be safely said that many Europeans were uncomfortable with the manner in which Greece was about to be pillaged again. It had already been plundered by wealthy tax evaders.

Nevertheless, the real villain of the piece and cast as a sort of smiling assassin was European Central Bank (ECB) president, Mario Draghi, who made his debut late in the picture.

The Greek audience was about to gain even more interest.

In conclusion, after thirty-eight of his own MPs had voted against the bailout deal, the Greek PM should have concentrated on clawing back some credibility and, to use one of our local idioms, tell the failed EU to 'whistle for their euros' and return Greece to the drachma where at least the Greek people would be masters of their own destiny. Greece is rich in ancient cultural history and the associated tourism will sustain as the chief economic component for thousands of years to come – long after oil has run out. Tsipras might have agreed to the 86 billion-euro bailout for the collapsing banks in 2015, but it will eventually be the Greek people themselves who will decide whether further fiscal obstacles can be overcome. After all, it's the failed European financial institutions that enabled this situation to occur in the first place.

In the meantime, perhaps Tsipras should have gone one further in not adhering to EU protocol when refusing to wear a tie for conferences and suchlike and reverted to a more refined proletariat gesture. Instead of waving the white flag, sticking two fingers up to Angela Merkel and the discredited European Union would have been a much more effective semaphore.

The Foreign Legions

Only two English players, in Butland and Johnson (both being recent acquisitions to the first team), in the Stoke City line-up against Leicester City during the 2015–16 Premier League season was not good enough. Yes, it's nice to see a little international flair in English football, yet the overseas player influx has increased to such an extent that good English players now struggle to come through. Today, in 2018, foreign line-ups are representative of most Premier League clubs with many fans saying that it's not English football any more. I remember in the late 1970s when foreign imports were sparse. We had the Argentinian duo of Osvaldo Ardiles and Ricardo Villa who played for Spurs and locally the Dutch midfielder, Loek Ursem, became the first 'imported' signing for Stoke City in 1979. The theory goes that one can buy better quality for less capital on the external market and that is the main reason we have seen the slow demise of the English player. Alternatively, others would advocate that it can be even more cost-effective nurturing talent at home. Such was/is the continental dominance of the 'English' Premier League, inevitably it is only the better continental players who will be highlighted and promoted and as so, will have the best chance of advancing. The same goes with English club managers. Out of the twenty clubs in the Premier League going into the season 2018–19, there are only four English managers compared with seventeen, twenty years ago. Are you seriously telling me that our English managers aren't as gifted as their foreign counterparts?

What the Dickens

I must say that I do fancy myself as a bit of a culture vulture at times. The Dickens Museum at 48–49 Doughty Street, London, WC1N 2LX can provide one with an interesting historical, cultural and literary perspective on the life of Charles Dickens.

The Costumed Tour is a must.

The museum itself is within walking distance of London Euston and King's Cross railway stations (taking a right onto Guilford Street from Gray's Inn Road and then taking the first left onto Doughty Street); it takes about fifteen minutes from King's Cross. In the King's Cross/St. Pancras vicinity one might have to ask for directions (if you struggle with the North and South directives on Google Maps like I do). Still, on the plus side, this can be an opportunity to meet real Londoners. I enjoy playing 'Spot the Londoner' and any subsequent interactions that might ensue when asking for directions is a bonus, especially if you like the accent, as I do. The vast majority of locals go out of their way to guide you to your destination (nowadays via their mobile phones). If you are looking for a more obscure destination (like the Dickens Museum) nipping into a shop is a favoured idea as they will more often than not harbour some local knowledge.

Apparently, the museum is the actual house where Charles Dickens lived from 1837 until 1839. He wrote *Oliver Twist* and *Nicholas Nickleby* while resident there. I was so relieved that I had opted for the Costumed Tour (a few pounds extra) for when the housemaid opened the door to greet us we knew we were in for a treat of a different kind. Going into themed mode playing the part of the subservient servant but honoured to be the housemaid of someone of notable personage, the period enactment was engrossing, to say the least. In character and assuming the demeanour of the time (graced with the authentic accentuated tongue – and lots of it) the maid began to show us around Dickens' house as if he still lived there; educating us to boot.

The house design (including furnishings) is thought to be exactly the same as it was in 1839. So as not to spoil it for others who wish to visit the museum, I will relay only a couple of factual titbits regarding the tour. One is that Dickens' father was imprisoned for bad debts and two, hedgehogs were kept downstairs in many Victorian kitchens to eat the many insects that thrived there.

The Dissolution of the Union

Who would have thought that, after the Scottish referendum on independence in September 2014, where a 'No' vote prevailed, just months later the 'UK' general election would see the SNP (Scottish National Party) emerge as a commanding political force in the whole of the 'UK'.

Did any of our political know-alls at the BBC see that one coming post-referendum?

In effect, and without signing any proclamation to rubber stamp the implication, Scotland has separated from England and has all but become an independent entity. Yes, the May 7th 2015 general election might not have been a platform for the Scottish independence question, still, the SNP's ideological and political core is based on the premise of autonomy for Scotland and the Scottish people voted for that same SNP.

Strange how things come full circle, isn't it?

The big twist to this fascinating British Islands political saga is that the focus will no doubt eventually switch to English independence. For too long England has carried the weight of the home nations of Scotland, Wales, and Ireland like monkeys on her back.

Latent English nationalism is inherent within the English conscious and unconscious mind which could eventually materialise into self-sufficiency for England as one of four independent countries assembled under one cooperative British islands umbrella. Maybe the Union has already begun to dissolve within the deep recesses of the British political psyche. After all, as we edge toward the year 2019, many would agree that the cement holding the union together is beginning to crack and crumble.

Can English separatists now begin to organise? The central social principles as ascribed to compassionate governance, coupled with a withdrawal from the current European Union and strict immigration controls as add-ons, would further the English sovereignty appeal. An attractive, dynamic, fair and free market economy/business structure could also be a key feature in attracting voters to a new English Party for English people.

In saying that, the ideological strata with which to flesh out a new English National Party would be England's separation from the adjoining 'UK' states of Scotland, Wales and Northern Ireland. After all, why passively wait for those said states to secede from us?

An original English dominion would have mass appeal which would see England still remaining one of the richest countries in the world. An independent England would also be the biggest and most populous of the home nations, it would still command respect and importance on a global scale and would remain an important financial centre. After all, throughout time our country had always been known as the Independent Kingdom of England until the Act of Union in 1707.

In the event of English self-government there would be no need to adopt the West Lothian Question of English votes for English laws. There would also be no need for the unequal Barnett formula either.

There is some credence in the reports that the English resented the prospect of a Scottish (SNP) involvement (in an arrangement with Labour) in some sort of Westminster administration. The Scots will not take this personally though; this resentment will only reinforce their positional identity and assertion that there are fundamental differences within the home nations' framework which would enable them all to fare better as separate identities.

Nonetheless, post-election 2015, the sick, the low-paid, together with the majority of the UK population battened down their hatches in anticipation of an austerity bombardment like never seen before. The Tories didn't disappoint. The attack on the vulnerable and the services the vulnerable need to live a dignified life, rained down hard and fast, with a cruelty unimagined and over a sustained period of time. Those said Tory bullies who had a licence to inflict suffering on the populace as never seen before showed little mercy.

In this event, the SNP will not necessarily have to look for a material change like the 'UK' government voting to opt out of the European Union to call another referendum. After three or four more years subjected to this brand of Tory rule the majority of the Scottish electorate will be begging for independence whatever devolved sweeteners are afforded them in lieu.

On a more positive note, the remarkable general election of May 7th, 2015, saw the likes of Danny Alexander and the Lib Dem charlatans wiped off the political landscape and no, they won't recover.

Lest we never forget: Tuition Fees, Tuition Fees, Tuition Fees.

Turning back to England, career politicians who openly decry those who aspire to be free to self-determine their own political/geographical futures, to quote an old English word, will always be exposed to hreowan (rue) the day.

There is a climate to facilitate the need for irrevocable political/geographical change on these islands.

Notes: the SNP lost seats in the 2017 general election, the thinking being that the electorate voted on the independence question. The SNP (for Scottish independence) gained thirty-five seats and the Conservative/Labour/Lib Dem (Unionist Coalition) gained twenty-four seats. This means that there is now a clear majority for Scottish independence, not the opposite, like the pro-unionist camps like to infer.

It's now all about timing.

Engineering Genius at the Etruria Industrial Museum

It is difficult to define a genius. Conjointly, the genius has only been found in the upper echelons of society in the historical scheme of things. Let's face it – it would have been difficult to discover an engineering virtuoso on the factory floors of England over the centuries. If there were any; they wouldn't have been acknowledged.

Alternatively, true genius is not necessarily found within the realms of privilege because that same status would have allowed 'the genius' to conduct expensive research and forge the right connections for their genius to materialise into invention or publication. The true definition of a genius, therefore, is more likely to be the individual with mental or emotional difficulties intertwined with a supreme intellect and from a lower educational background.

What's the phrase: 'There is a fine line between insanity and genius'?

Some believe that true genius is also found in those that are not aware of it; so in not being sentient of their own capabilities, the scholarly threads of their inner thought processes naturally syphon off compliments or adulation. In turn, this allows that same intellect to expand enough to allow probes of other 'outside the box' theories and alternative equations to what is conventionally accepted.

Subjectively speaking, the most innovative and exciting inventions have been the aircraft, the word processor, the radio signal and the process of photography invented by Louis Daguerre (1787–1851).

On a visit to the Etruria Industrial Museum and Heritage Centre recently

I pondered on the notion of the technical genius. Not being bothered to fix a plug myself, it was most interesting to contemplate how such a light matter like steam can propel heavy apparatus, keeping in mind of course that the complex machinery as seen at the museum was state of the art in its day.

Then we have James Brindley (1716–72) to whom a statue is dedicated alongside the Trent and Mersey canal, which is adjacent to the Industrial Museum. Was he ingenious in his sphere? Born into an advantaged family in Derbyshire but spending most of his life in Leek, Staffordshire, he became one of the most noted engineers of his epoch and the inspiration behind the first canal construction.

But would he have been such a notable genius if he were not born into a well-to-do family?

No he wouldn't. But that's not the point.

Genius aside, a visit to the Etruria Industrial Museum and Heritage Centre proffers a much broader industrial education than just the mechanisms surrounding a steam-powered potter's mill. As well as being able to witness the blacksmith at work, we also learn that the factory/ museum was hit by German bombers during the Second World War (the shells were intended for the massive steel works at nearby Shelton Bar).

We also discover at the museum that those who like to exude sophistication by ingesting tea from a nice expensive bone china cup would think again. For all intents and purposes, one is in reality sipping from a receptacle made from refined animal bones and flint.

To think; this is in common with ancient human beings living in the south of England towards the end of the last ice age who made human skulls into drinking vessels, according to Dr Silvia Bello of the London Natural History Museum.

Animal bone is animal bone, you know.

Well, let's forget the above educational titbit for now and concentrate on the point of the article.

Because of cuts by the council, the Etruria Industrial Museum and Heritage Centre's opening times are variable (2018).

This is a travesty, taking on board the stimulating education the museum can offer our budding technical and engineering experts of the future.

In saying that, can't councils subsidise the museum via the education sector or from another funding body, so a visit to Etruria can be included in the school, college or university curriculum?

After all, the word engineering is a derivative of the Latin words *ingenium*, which means 'cleverness', and *ingeniare*, which means 'to devise'.

Proficient local engineers are a natural prerequisite for any forward-thinking city.

The law of averages states that eventually, and through the ordinary classes, we will then produce that rare creature called the humble genius.

England's World Cup Glory 2018

The World Cup staged in Russia in June and July 2018 has thrown out some interesting trivia. With regard to Russia generally, my observations when visiting, as seen in the article *Dispelling those Moscow Myths*, have been reinforced – not just by England fans visiting the biggest country on earth, but by the wider world. Hence, it was reprehensible that the English were put off visiting Russia because of unprecedented media vitriol (even by their sad standards) and missed a marvellous, uplifting, once-in-a generation sporting event as a consequence.

Even though sporting nationalism is an important and prideful sensation (yes, a few did get a tad carried away). If we really want to feature in the final of 2022, we must recognise the sad fact that England had easy pairings in the 2018 tournament and once they did come up against credible opposition (Croatia) they folded.

Yes, as a national team we are below par.

Yet, the great international success for the Russians and the English alike (Russia made the quarter-finals themselves) did not deter the 'UK' government from re-entering political fantasy mode. Apparently, the nerve agent Novichok had been confirmed in poor old embattled and beleaguered Wiltshire once again (July 5th) just six days before England's semi-final showdown with Croatia. Furthermore, it was all down to those dastardly ex-Soviets and ongoing investigations could last for months (in other words the powers that be can drip feed us this drivel for weeks to come). It appears that the establishment was not happy with the World Cup being a success. Parallel to the Novichok conspiracy, on the 9th July 2018, Sky News reported that the Royal Navy was to increase its presence in the North Atlantic because of the Russian threat. It almost imbecilic, isn't it?

As for the England team, let's hope their achievement this time around in the World Cup did not just mean success for the giant corporations. Will some of the millions generated from England's unlikely progression be channelled towards football academies (especially in under-privileged English towns), so our youth stand a fair chance of competing in the glutted-with-foreign-players Premier League?

Probably not.

Footnote: The eventual winners 'France' gained world-wide recognition for another conundrum: More than half of the French squad can trace their ancestry back to Africa.

Therefore, were Africa the real 2018 World Cup winners?

Situations Vacant:
Red Herring Catcher

One wonders where all the so-called jobs are for those out of work; the jobs just aren't there. Job clubs appear to be latest gimmick adopted by the DWP, where, at these centres, benefit claimants are forced to actively engage with DWP overseers in order to find work and if they aren't 'eager beaver enough' and slack off, they could be sanctioned (their benefits stopped indefinitely).

Not so long ago, the government's mandate seemed to come from the general populace who used to resent those on benefits, but that seems to be changing (2018).

Most of us will need to rely on some kind of benefit at some point in our lives. So in effect, the general public are doing themselves out of their own future benefits if they devoutly believe in benefit cuts. A free TV licence for senior citizens is a benefit, isn't it?

Previous schemes like the Permitted Work Scheme (2013) should have advertised for a 'red herring catcher' in their situations vacant column. This would have cut to the chase. The red herring is easily identifiable in this equation because although those on ESA could do only some permitted work of less than sixteen hours per week and earn £97.50 on top of their benefits, many employers did not advertise jobs of less than sixteen hours per week and the ones that were on offer were low-paid and menial. Are those on Jobseeker's Allowance therefore no more than a malleable reserve workforce. As in, when the multinational has exhausted and privatised one institution, they can move on to another when the 'economy' picks up. Thus, having a ready and able workforce on very little money, ready to fill that labour gap once again – and so the capitalist cycle to work idea neverendingly circles.

Voluntary work is a better option for others out of work, although volunteers have to be careful of not being used to do the jobs others in the same company refuse to do. Well at least if one fills a voluntary post and it does not suit and one quits, benefits won't be stopped (you hope); even though one has filled out a lengthy application form for an unpaid job. Then we have those disabled, who are terrified to undertake voluntary work just in case their disability benefits are cut.

As for Universal Credit, the idea that the DWP pay housing benefit directly to the claimant and not to the landlord suggests that the government are either incompetent or are purposely initiating social upheaval.

Talk about the Third World; is there such thing as a Fourth?

Pain and the Isolation Ward

There is nothing like fly on the wall reporting, whereas, the writer is part of the events unfolding and has first-hand knowledge of those occurrences. This does not necessarily equate to the writer documenting the incidents in secret. It is about documenting events factually and accurately. I made no secret of the fact I was documenting my experiences at the University Hospital of North Staffordshire (now The Royal Stoke University Hospital) a few years back. My real life experience started with Accident and Emergency (A&E) which was visited at approximately 1pm on 24/9/2013 because of chronic pain in my kidney area. After waiting over an hour in reception, a consultant shouted me through and I was then seen by a doctor who heard my complaint. Instructed to give a urine sample, it was then relayed that I would need my bladder to be full if I were to undergo further tests. All they could offer was paracetamol for pain relief.

Another doctor then came to me and asked me to relay the same story, to which I explained that the story had already been told once and it should have been recorded as notes. I was then instructed to drink water to fill my bladder up again because blood had been found in my urine and a scan was therefore required.

When my bladder was full after drinking water, I was taken to the Clinical Decision Unit (CDU) which was quite a long way off from X-ray and so had to sit in uncomfortable pain waiting to be scanned. It almost seemed farcical when X-ray staff asked me my name and date of birth "just in case they had not got the right one". Then, after the scan, I was misdirected by a staff member back to the CDU where, when I found it, I was allocated a sort of 'medical holding cell' to await further decisions.

At the CDU there was no communal facility in which one could occupy oneself with TV or the internet. There was also no apparatus to make tea or coffee or to interact with other patients. This facility was almost like being jailed.

A dementia patient was also wandering around the area, obviously distressed at being held in one of the 'cells'.

After hours had gone by, held in the CDU unit in that one room, I ventured out into the corridor to see other human life. It was most shocking when a senior staff member then asked me if I would go back into my room because they wanted to discuss confidential information.

After feeling belittled by this request, I stated that my personal details should not be discussed in a corridor at the main desk. I suggested they go into a back room to discuss confidential matters concerning patients. The seemingly overworked staff member in question accepted the point I had made but the damage had been done.

Approximately seven hours after my initial contact with the hospital (at around 8pm) and after constant requests for an update regarding my situation, a doctor came to see me and asked the same questions as the other two doctors (had I been vomiting, feeling pain, passing water, etcetera). The eventual grim tidings were that I had a cystic mass on my kidney, together with a large kidney stone that could not pass naturally. I naturally asked if the cystic growth was dangerous, with the doctor responding that further tests like ultrasound would need to be undertaken to ascertain these facts.

A nurse later informed me, while taking my blood and fitting me up with a drip, that cysts can become tumours; I did not know if I had been given a possible death sentence or not and went into mild shock, owing to the fact that it could possibly be curtains for 'Controversial Kev'. (The word controversy is almost controversial in itself. Controversial means disputable, debateable or contentious. Facts and truth are never up for dispute, although it is accepted that truth can be subjective).

After being given a meal that would not feed a sparrow, I was admitted to the Surgical Assessment Unit (SAU) in the Lyme Building where another doctor pointed out to me in more detail that many patients had cysts, alongside kidney stones, which were usually benign. This made me feel more optimistic although I would have to await further tests for confirmation.

At this interval it should be pointed out that I was/am aware that there are caring professionals employed by the NHS who are possibly operating under a fractured system. Others fob you off when asking them questions about your situation with the standard 'I will find out' or they need to tend to a more urgent patient first. I argued that every patient's situation is subjective to themselves; and although patients are cognisant that there are others in a more serious condition, their own condition always takes precedence.

Spending the night hospitalised, the very next day it was noted that mealtimes in hospital are so officious it is reminiscent of the Florence Nightingale era. Food is despatched in a regimented fashion at designated times, accompanied by one standard half cup of tea and that is that. On the SAU there was a lack of pillows and you had to walk to the bathroom holding that long stick that your drip was attached to. More elderly patients, who had to repeatedly visit the bathroom because of bladder problems, were expected to undertake this deed too. Blood pressure and temperature tests also had to be taken every hour, which seemed more like a precaution against possible legal claims than looking after the patient. Surely, blood pressure tests should only be administered to patients that need them most and the resources shifted to managing the doctors.

In the morning, after a bad night's sleep, an 'unknown group' accompanied by a doctor came around my bed to inform me that an ultrasound would be needed because, although they thought I had got a cyst, they needed to be sure because the X-ray image was not good for looking for cysts.

I started to become alarmed again. It was then relayed that there is a special machine for breaking up kidney stones but it is not always available. While waiting for my ultrasound results other patients told me their stories. One man had been suffering a rumbling appendix for some four days and had still not been operated on. Another had gallstones and his medication had been waylaid. In addition, another patient was repeatedly going for the same test. Surely in many cases it is better for the patient to manage their pain at home and free the bed up for a more deserving case.

It was quite apparent that the most serious concern for patients (myself included) was the 'waiting game' as in you just sit or lie there for hours waiting for news from the doctors. At approximately 4pm I received the news from another doctor (after seeing some five different doctors in all) that my cyst was definitely benign and I would return to the hospital in four weeks after taking tablets to loosen the tube (through which my stone had a 40% chance of passing naturally). It was further explained that if the stone was still there after one month I would have to undergo keyhole surgery to remove it.

Yours truly then came to the conclusion that the governing NHS protocol was to cover every option other than to perform invasive surgery. I did not believe that this policy was in place to save the patient distress but more about saving money.

Travelling Backwards in London

Having already documented the crushes on the London Midland train from London Euston to Crewe, for my endeavours I was placated with a cheap free ticket. Hence, it might be prudent to take on-board what I am saying before there is a serious accident, where commuters could be crushed on the trains and tubes in London, especially during rush hour. In addition, only God knows how those with a fear of closed spaces fare – they obviously cannot travel during peak footfall periods, which has legal ramifications under disability laws.

London should be projected as a proud, forward-thinking metropolis with a rapid comfortable transport system for all, not by the 'Capital of Backward Britain' tag currently ascribed to it. Then there are the injurious gases given out by the buses – and the time it takes to cross the system on the contraptions, but that's another piece. That same piece could be marketed as a new tourist attraction called 'Going Backwards on the Buses'.

If this situation wasn't so serious it would be comical.

On April 27th 2017, at around 8am, I watched with my own eyes how they were packing people onto Great Northern trains at Palmers Green; on trains that appeared more like dangerous cattle trucks, to put it bluntly. As for Sadiq Khan, Mayor of London; yes, ivory towers are at great distance from the realities of what the masses have to suffer at ground level on a daily basis. Besides, elected representatives have a responsibility to initiate something more than cosmetic exercises or vanity projects. I eventually squeezed on to a Great Northern train bound for Finsbury Park. I then changed at Finsbury Park for a tube to Euston but had to leave the train at Highbury and Islington because I could hardly breathe due to overpacked compartments.

I then watched about twelve tube trains go past bound for Brixton, all so ram-jam-packed, it would have been foolish to board. There was a gentleman crushed up with his back to the tube who nearly got his head stuck in the closing door. This was seen with my own eyes.

Eventually braving the crush, I pondered as to what would happen in the event of an accident, as in there would be nowhere to escape to; I tried to imagine the suffocating horror.

Something needs to be initiated with immediate effect to address this disgraceful and maladroit London Transport situation. All stops should be pulled out if we are to maintain London's position on the economic stage (and as an attractive tourist destination). If this transport chaos perpetuates unchallenged, our capital will eventually be known to future generations as the evanescent financial capital.

Yes, it's that bad.

Backdrop to the
Tunisian Narrative

Having visited many tourist destinations worldwide, I most definitely struck an affinity with the Tunisian resort of Sousse. So much so that I have holidayed there twice. Only a two-and-a-half-hour flight from East Midlands/Manchester/Birmingham to Monastir, the sun could be guaranteed from March through to November.

Always mindful of the geopolitical climate, even though the last time I had visited had been some thirteen years previous (staying at the Marhaba hotel on that occasion), it did not go unnoticed that on the world map, Tunisia is sandwiched in between the Islamic hotbeds of Algeria and Libya.

Yet, it was some eight years ago that I came to the decision that Tunisia was out of bounds and off the world map for me personally. This was due to that same volatile political climate that affects the whole of North Africa, including Morocco and Egypt. Which brings me on to Prime Minister of the time David Cameron's assertion that the atrocity perpetrated on the beaches of Sousse on the 26th June 2015, that left thirty-eight dead (including thirty Britons and three Irish citizens) could happen anywhere in the world. Yes, this sort of outrage can happen anywhere in the world, but you will raise your chances of being caught up in such atrocities by holidaying in North Africa.

Furthermore, how do the West and her allies propose to eradicate the perennial ISIS threat – by closing down mosques and/or introducing armed guards at holiday hotspots? And what will the British government do in response to the recent massacre; despatch some 'removed from real life' anti-terrorist specialist to liaise with other experts in the field? Or maybe the Cobra meetings initiated in the aftermath of the bloodbath will conclude with a response to invade Tunisia just like they did Iraq?

I did note whilst on holiday in Sousse that there is great poverty. The multitudinous poor rely on the tourists for survival and if Tunisian males can strike a relationship with an older visitor (of either sex) they have hit the jackpot.

We called her the fifty-year-old; a middle-aged English lady who had become involved in a romantic relationship with a young handsome twenty-eight-year-old Tunisian. When she flounced into the hotel like a loved-up teenager all heads would turn. She had hit the jackpot too.

I can also remember walking out of the Marhaba hotel onto the road outside where the 'nippers' used to sit. Yes, such was their animal guile (most likely down to not knowing where their next meal was coming from) they would know you were outside of the hotel grounds before you did. Some thirteen years ago local Tunisians were excluded from the hotels and the beaches those same hotels presided over. I could not help feeling that deep down the locals detested us but relied on us to survive. I remember one English holidaymaker declaring that the local currency, the dinar, "was their God".

Then there was the incident with the hotel activities coordinator who I had spotted outside of the hotel complex, although he was difficult to recognise. The reason being because the hotel employee was not smiling. When he noticed us, the contrived grin reappeared on cue. In other words, he had been briefed to 'smile at the tourists' at all costs.

The best thing about Sousse, besides the fabulous jet skis and quad bike safari trips, was the camaraderie between the British compatriots at the hotels. It was so easy to make friends. There was old Bob. from Newcastle-upon-Tyne. who told stories of what it was like gambling in the back streets of Newcastle before the bookies started up. Then there was the Irish girl, Claire. Who relayed that she felt something was not quite right with Tunisia and I knew exactly what she meant.

Most of us from the home nations treated the locals in Sousse with the utmost respect. Regardless, there were those who saw the natives as slave-like. I can recall how I used to scoff at some of the guests for dressing up in their finery for the three-star evening meal that could feature hairy fish (I used to go vegetarian when in Tunisia). I vividly recall one German lady sitting in the reception area trussed up and fluttering a fan, very colonial-like, as she waited for the clock to strike six (which would signify that dinner would be served, the highlight of the day for many).

I also remember when one of the hotel chefs joined us at a nearby bar and 'John' (a middle-aged/elderly Scottish gentleman) had slapped the chef across the face to demonstrate he could just do whatever he liked to the locals and they could do nothing about it. John was a big fish in a small pond and he had something that the Tunisians didn't have – money.

Then there was the occasion when we visited the Medina market in Sousse. Taxis were cheap and the market was only a short car ride from the hotel area.

Some young guys were selling leather jackets for £5 in one shop. Of course it was a sales gimmick and they turned mockingly aggressive when we cottoned on. When I asked my friend what she would have done if the jackets were really priced at £5 she replied that she would have ordered a fleet of taxis to ferry stacks of the jackets back to the hotel.

And the Medina stallholders thought they were ruthless.

The moral of this story lies in the backdrop narrative which tries to inform regarding real relationships between the Tunisians and British holidaymakers in the resort of Sousse. Whether or not that resort will ever recover from the merciless slayings of those nice, decent and, most of all, innocent, British people on June 26th remains to be seen. This, in turn, poses the question; will tourists ever feel safe enough to return?

Does the answer to this question lie in another question? As in, will we ever feel safe wherever we are as long as there are Western interferences in Afghanistan, Syria, Libya and Iraq?

If the expropriation of natural resources in the Middle East is not responsible for the carnage seen in recent years, can someone tell me what is?

The Romans were Taking the Pee

Anxiety is a complex mental health problem for many people and can feel like varying degrees of fear. Like fixation, anxiety, when linked to something we are fixating about, has an overpowering premise in wanting to maintain that state of fear by having us stewing and over-analysing what is/was making us catastrophise, which can see our overall mental state worsening. Why would our brain allow us to constantly dwell on what is making us anxious, one asks? This is because the brain is unwell and is malfunctioning, which, in turn, can manifest into physical symptoms like sweating and shaking. Anxiety uses any vehicle (life events, for example) to attach itself to, in order to traumatise, so you can either opt to sit in it or you can choose to dilute it. Dwelling on issues connected to a recent bereavement beset with experiencing severe fear, I not only engaged with bereavement counselling which was very productive, but also chose to take a trip to Avon and Somerset (or should I say, Bath and North-East Somerset, or is it Bristol, North Somerset and South Gloucestershire – ridiculous isn't it?).

After visiting Taunton in autumn (no cider jokes please), I headed for Bristol Temple Meads railway station (built in 1840) to take the eleven-minute train journey to Bath. Isn't it most odd why only Bath has something deep inside the earth's core that heats up water into hot springs. In Bath, Mendip Hills rain water saturates the limestone where geothermal energy then heats up the H2O.

It was the Celts who first utilised the hot springs and dedicated them to the Goddess Sulis. But like so many times in history, Roman propaganda pervaded to paint the ancient English as backward barbaric savages (that's propaganda folks) who did not possess the intellect or resources to recognise such a natural wonder.

According to our modern-day historians, who have regurgitated the nonsense, the indigenous Backward Betties only used the hot springs to dip their pigs into.

Back to the present, (the Roman Baths) on entering, I encountered a mysterious soothsayer lady sitting by the spring, attired in Roman costume of the times. I sat down next to her to engage with the act, which cued the old crone to ask me if I would like a bed for the night with straw and dormouse for supper. Of course, most of us know the Romans ate mice, but wash their clothes in human urine? Never. The lady then expanded on how the Romans gargled with urine, used it to soothe stings (which is logical because of the ammonia) and even imported a spicy Portuguese variety in large vats.

After asking a very pleasant Spanish tourist to take some snaps of me, I wished I hadn't. How could I doctor those coarse monkey-skin flap (jowl) lines as seen on both cheeks, I considered? Those waters weren't going to shift that age-related deformity any day soon, therapeutic properties or no therapeutic properties; even if I dipped my head in the spring for a month.

Did the Romans have a derivative of Botox? They seemed to have an answer for everything else.

Age does keep recurring throughout these chronicles, doesn't it? Perhaps it's because seeing oneself age is parallel to witnessing a wicked disfiguring shadow of your former self. I should be thankful I am not completely grey – oh God, that's to come.

Every picture tells a different story though, shopping therapy in the beautiful Georgian city of Bath can make one forget one's ageing boat race. When I tried on some new togs in-store, the reflection when posing in the mirror was a little more pleasing, monkey-skin flap-wise that is. In recognition of my new-found presence, the shop assistants sort of milled around with a little extra vim, especially when I politely declared, Caesar-like, that I would like any garment in air force blue.

Perhaps those two cartons of warm spring water I had gulped down at the Roman Baths ten minutes previously had done the trick.

The Big Alcohol Debate

The Big Alcohol Debate (in conjunction with Healthwatch Stoke-on-Trent) held at the Jubilee Hall in Stoke was, by and large, an interesting event. The debate also coincided with Alcohol Awareness Week.

The deliberation also featured a panel of experts coupled with performances by New Vic Borderlines, who interspersed the discourse by enacting real-life scenarios portraying those troubled by alcohol.

Considering that the majority of all crime reported today is substance-related, Staffordshire Police opened up the debate by expanding on the escalation of 'preloading', where people were getting drunk at home before hitting the town centres. Although currently causing all sorts of problems this practice is not new; many engaged in preloading or 'a few liveners' before going out some thirty-five years ago.

The police representative did outline a possible shock-tactics pilot scheme which could include videoing those carousing drunkenly on the pub and club scene. There would then be a follow-up visit by health professionals the morning after to show the perpetrator their own embarrassing footage.

This prospective measure appeared to be a very positive step forward in addressing the 'too drunk to stand' crisis affecting young people at the weekends. The reason why Britain is one of the few European countries where alcohol inebriation leads to weekend mayhem in our town centres is also most odd.

Young women are thought to be vulnerable in our town centres, often getting estranged from their friends due to over-intoxication, which can sometimes result in serious corollaries.

What is more, sexual improprieties sometimes committed by both males and females while under the influence could affect them in the long run, both physically (with sexually transmitted diseases) and psychologically (it is believed that casual sex can engender serious long-term emotional issues).

The tabled parties then enabled sensible discussion around alcohol problems where a facilitator summed up the respective group discussions for the collective audience.

Our table examined advertising and the availability of alcohol, which was by all accounts thought to be dressed up as a must-have commodity. Moreover, when a representative from the council asked us to concentrate on the local perspective it was pointed out that this was difficult due to the fact that it was the multinational supermarkets selling brand names who were, by and large, the main merchandisers locally.

Industrial heritage and social conditions were also discussed, as in it was believed that potters in the area escaped the torment and servitude of everyday working life in the 19th and 20th centuries by resorting to alcohol as an anaesthetic. The link was then made to social conditions of today and the expectations and pressures put on people by conventional societal demands which were also thought to be linked to alcohol addiction.

Educating children from a very young age was also thought to be key to changing the culture of alcohol consumption.

There seemed to be a general consensus that statements like 'one or two drinks can be good for you' were misleading and dangerous as already expanded on in a previous article. The group was unanimous in believing that alcohol is a mind-altering drug and can cause more devastation than many of the other available narcotics around and should be treated as such. Imagine the furore, if those same addiction 'experts' who govern the services associated with substance misuse advocated that it is okay to have one or two tokes of the crack pipe.

The practical side of the event saw the first routine by New Vic Borderlines portraying a middle-class type in denial, in that there was no more room left in her wheelie bin for general waste because her wine bottle empties had rendered it full to the brim. The second routine contradicted the cultural notion that it is comical to be drunk. This was exemplified by a young man making an idiot of himself complete with the distinct bog-standard wet patch appropriated to his crotch.

The questions and answer session began soon after with the spokesperson from every table posing a question to the panel.

It appeared that there seemed to be a lack of understanding at times from certain members of the panel, especially with regard to the notion of reducing alcohol strength to combat problematic imbibing. Those who work in the addiction sphere know too well that if people want to get drunk or 'hit the spot' they will manage it whatever the strength of the liquor.

Furthermore, some of the panel members only seemed to have a theoretical understanding of the insights regarding irremediable addiction struggles. One such member exemplified the point that measures were being implemented to offset the drinking scourge by stating that the dangerously potent White Lightning cider had been withdrawn from the shelves. What was not expanded on was that there are many equivalents now taking its place.

One question put to the panel asked whether Stoke-on-Trent is monitoring the strategies used by Newcastle-under-Lyme in that the borough is making some incursions into the social epidemic (even though there is a long way to go) by sensible policing and initiating first aid marquees in the town centre at weekends to take the pressure off A&E.

The police spokesperson on the panel responded by saying that they were watching Newcastle very closely.

Although there were many interesting questions in between, the last question focused on the criminal justice/prison system, whereby many recidivists are alcohol- or substance-dependent.

The underlying message from this question centred on the fact that there are many in need of support to survive what life throws at them without resorting to alcohol.

In conclusion, the information disseminated from the Big Alcohol Debate was that our local institutions and governing bodies need to tap into the views and experiences of those who have lived experience of self-destructing during their desperate personal battles with the demon drink.

Non-textbook real-life stories are always the most informative.

Controlling Infatuation One Way

When involved in the mating game the rules of that game are anything but fair. Take infatuation, for example. The realities are that the cocktail of chemicals and neurological changes at play when engulfed by infatuation, coupled with reduced serotonin levels (which is thought to regulate emotion), makes for a heady mix. Not forgetting, of course, that when seduced by the infatuated state, the frontal cortex closes down so you are blind to any faults that the focus of your attention may or may not have.

Yes, you're on dangerous ground.

It can start innocuously, by simply liking another person, to progressing into being held spellbound by their pheromones. Yes, we have discovered that they secrete that magical, biological, attracting-you formula that others do not. Furthermore, some become attracted to that same person very quickly because they meet a deep unconscious primordial need. Their type is compatible with our DNA code.

Then, for many, I'm afraid, it morphs into a horrendous preoccupation where territoriality enters the amalgam. Now deluded, those besotted oddly believe that the object (as they will be referred to in this piece) is their property, and as a result, become insanely jealous at the mere thought of others 'breaching their patch'. This jealousy is best described as a chronic tension, emanating from the deep, anxious pit of the gut, whirring never-endingly at the thought of anyone else gaining access to their domain. Naked sexual attraction is a powerful and destructive force, perpetuated by fear-based adrenaline, pumped by the desire for exclusivity with that particular object. Infatuation is about your need for ownership or control of the person; the irony being that you are the one being controlled.

Irrational behaviour is also commonplace when overpowered by the purgatorial infatuated state. You painstakingly plot your 'contact them' modus operandi for hours on end, by going over the same script as to why you should not hurriedly connect with the focus of your desire, but to find yourself collapsing and doing the exact opposite (making contact too soon) sometimes within seconds, without even thinking about it, such is the command the infatuation has over your very being.

The truth is, you don't look forward to texts from your object; you agonisingly wait for them for the whole day. And what a disappointment when you hear the beep of your phone to discover it is only 'Aunty Florrie' and not the focus of your desire. Other loved ones have become unimportant and secondary when engrossed in your smitten state.

Don't despair though, the experts conclude that, such is your unhinged state of mind when infatuated, scientific analysis as to why you repeatedly go over the same terrain of 'what ifs' concerning scenarios past, present, and future in relation to your object will eventually be identified as something more profound than OCD or rumination.

No doubt you also correspond or associate most things you see and hear (like place names or songs) with that same person which can, in turn, trigger abdominal nervous tension. You also imagine being at the dinner table, for example, playing out the part of entertaining your object-of-desire's family, even though you have only engaged in just one or two innocent dates.

What's more, other doyens in the field reckon your powerful attraction holds the same composites to that of taking cocaine. One interviewed subject stated that when their object called off a prospective rendezvous (cut off the supply) they moaned like a wounded animal. Subsequently, that same subject then reverted to plan B, which was to meet another person they did not deem as attractive, so they could gratify the craving in some small way, shape or form. Notwithstanding, they described this demotion as a mental wellbeing dégringolade on a par with taking Bolivian Flake (their infatuation) to ingesting street Speed (plan B).

Then we have limerence, which is apparently a prolonged intense infatuation with added strength of desire (God help them is all I can say).

Limerent or not, you can draw up battle plans to counteract your, by now, manic infatuated state. You can look for another love interest to dilute, discuss with a trustworthy sounding board, you can self-analyse your own shortcomings, concentrate on your intended's negatives, or more dramatically, you can put an elastic band on your wrist and tweak it to give you a biting sting every time your passion pops into mind (yes, you will wind up with one hell of a weal). Whatever you do, the object of your desire is not going to budge. Some even speculate that it's better to just purge the demon by wallowing in the grief (you know that deep down you just want to be alone with your infatuation) thereafter, treating the whole miserable episode as a pathetic human state at which you can laugh. At the end of the day it will pass (you hope). See it for what it is, or was: a base mammalian crush that has no place in any half-civilised human brain. You might even come to the conclusion that as long as you can still function to earn your corn, why not while away your free time staring into space yearning for somebody you will probably never have. It will burn itself out eventually – won't it?

The truth is, you can't imagine the infatuation burning out of what emotional intelligence you have left, can you? Because at this stage, you are only thinking of the person 95% of your waking hours – and for the other 5% of the time, your object is in the back of your mind, hovering and burdening like a lurking spectre.

You are in such an apprehensive heightened state (a perpetual high alert) you are in physical danger too. Your fight or flight response button is also locked down on repeat, fuelled by lustful imaginations regarding your next tryst. There's no hope for you at this interval, let's just say you're doomed.

But the release of dopamine in your tiny Neanderthal brain (whether conscious or unconscious) makes it all worthwhile, doesn't it? In reality, you don't experience pleasure from being trapped by this attraction; you feel distress. Your reproductive urge does not feel like an exhilarating, heart pounding, butterfly in the stomach, but a never-satiated open sore. On top of everything, you have unwittingly cleared your calendar to make yourself readily available 24/7 for your object of desire. Sad and embarrassing; ring any bells? Had it, haven't you? At this interval you have probably scared the object of your desire into running for the hills in any case; desperately presenting on a plate is hardly attractive, is it?

On the other hand, some enamoured by infatuation can subconsciously self-sabotage and bring any hope of a possible future relationship with their intended crashing to a premature end, because to cut it off quickly with bitter recriminations (or initiate their object to cut it off for them) appears to be the only way they can stop themselves from sinking deeper into the infatuation mire. Yes, perhaps, just perhaps, they can begin to get over it. In the event of your decision to tackle the infatuation head-on, deleting all referents (including images) relating to your object in the hope of lessening all reminders is good advice. Then, remove your object's number from your phone but don't delete it. Subsequently, your next move will be to store that number in a place that will take you at least fifteen minutes to retrieve. This will address the impulse you will be experiencing to text your object, thus by the time you have located the number to text them, the urge to contact will have had time to diminish. If you are determined to make that connection, spending fifteen minutes retrieving the number is the better option than to make an ass of yourself via email or social media, which you would have had to do if you had deleted the phone number. At this crisis you will have some serious withdrawal symptoms to look forward to. Let's just say, "Get your turkey done"; infatuation will only leave you when it, and only it, decides to do so. You don't control your infatuated state, your infatuated state controls you.

Notes regarding this phase: don't listen to that little voice in your head which repeatedly invents excuses for you to make contact with the object. Listen instead to your true voice of wisdom which is giving you multiple reasons as to why it is not a good idea to make that contact. If you haven't already brought the friendship or 'relationship' crashing down and the object contacts you; just ignore them or say you are committed elsewhere, only when you begin to get over the infatuation will you stand any chance of remaining friends. Nevertheless, the chances are that once the passion has subsided, you will not wish to stay friends – after all, you wanted the object to be your lover, didn't you, and in the dispossessed light of day, you probably wouldn't want them anyway. Their genetic code was your match; but take heart from the fact that their intellectual/character code was perhaps an enormous mismatch which would never have sustained long-term.

There is good news on the infatuation horizon, believe it or not; because that's what infatuation is, just an infatuation which has no real emotional substance. In other words, because the relationship was one-sided and devoid of any loving depth, it will be much easier to get over. The obsession and related suffering will either fade gradually or you will wake up one morning and it will be gone; your brain will have defecated the emotional waste. Don't be complacent though; you might feel relieved because the obsession has paled considerably, but for that nervous, painful, internal apprehension to return without warning and with a vengeance. The dreaded return could be triggered by a succession of events, like a disappointing experience with a new romantic interest, which sees you taking a step back by perusing data regarding your object on social media. Yes, you are still infatuated by them. As already stipulated; bin all visual referents and do not succumb to the temptation of checking what they are up to – it will hurt you even more, especially if they are now in a relationship with someone else.

Let's face it, you might have felt empty before your object of desire came into your life but you have swiftly come to the conclusion that emptiness is the preferred option.

Perhaps the obtuse meanings behind the infatuated conundrum lie in evolutionary conditioning over millions of years, which has seen us programmed to breed at any cost. In saying that, there must be a widespread aberration in the human emotional state to allow such misery to transpire when consumed by infatuation – it goes against the grain of the pleasurable benefits associated with procreation. Then we have the question as to what is occurring when one's lust, love, or infatuation is unrequited, in that why are we still obsessed when we know deep down that the object of our desire will never feel the same way? Would some argue that such is the drive to control another human being (so they are exclusively ours) the club over the head used by our ancestors to take them anyway (whether they liked it or not) in order to guarantee the continuation of the species is our instilled metaphorical primal urge today.

Are you Winnie?

Waiting at the bus stop opposite Stoke-on-Trent railway station triggered this story. A visitor had asked which bus to catch and the conversation expanded to me relaying details of our local history. Firstly, I reminded them that we have a bad press from the uneducated with many outsiders believing that only the backward bunch are truly native to the Potteries. I would then disclose to the visitor that North Staffordshire is in the Peak District, Stoke-on-Trent's fascinating industrial heritage is second to none and our unique phraseology is by far the most interesting and dialectically diverse of all.

Then of course the Wedgwood Museum, which encompasses 250 years of local history, would get a plug. Yes, behind Wedgwood Pottery, named after our own master potter Josiah Wedgwood, grandfather of Charles Darwin, there are real-life stories to be told.

I remember my interview for the position of tray packer at Susie Cooper Pottery on the grimy and heavily polluted Newcastle Street, which was and still is a busy thoroughfare in and out of Burslem. Susie was a well-known and well-respected designer according to my mum's best friend Maggie Clooney. Wedgwood Pottery continued to produce Susie's designs which included 'Black Fruits' and 'Glen Mist'. Wedgwood also sustained the production of the 'can' shape which Susie Cooper initially designed in 1958.

Mr Foulkes had said, "Kevin, have you any criminal convictions?"

I hesitated.

"Er, no..."

"You hesitated, Kevin, is there something you are not telling us?"

"Well, when I was twelve I found some cigarette coupons and did not hand them in."

Turning back to Susie's novel designs, being a troubled pimply-faced seventeen-year-old at the time one wasn't interested in can shapes or anything like. On my first day after a successful interview, I entered the mustard-coloured Crown Works in between Burslem and Middleport with some anxiety; I wasn't partial to hard physical graft. It can be recalled that my mum could not wait to tell the rest of the family in that proud working class cluck that, 'Kevin's working.'

Kevin was working, all right, but many would deem it slave labour. Eight until a quarter to five, five and a half days a week, all for £60. And no, £60 was not a lot of money in those days. Then, come Sunday, you would be getting ready to do it all again. My new-found wealth did allow me to acquire a maroon-coloured Vespa motor scooter on hire purchase which would shuttle me to the factory and back to save me catching a bus. Yes, be thankful for small mercies my ancestors would espouse.

The year was 1979 and as a family we had moved back to Stoke-on-Trent from Kinmel Bay in North Wales and now resided in a nice three-bedroom detached in Bradeley, a not unpleasant suburb of Burslem. After a few months into my new job my mum would proudly remark to any interested parties that Kevin got up on his own and got himself off to work, although in all honesty sometimes she did cut my snappin (make my sandwiches). I had seen my mother get my older brother off to work, which would be a stressful drama to say the least. He would not get out of bed. On the rare occasion my mum could be 'buzzed' (had overslept herself). In the winter months it was icy torment to be the first one up and subsequently the first one downstairs to turn the gas fire on to defrost that early morning freeze.

My mother was an astute matriarchal figure, smart, nice of features and intermittently slightly rotund. She ruled the roost in-house. By contrast, my father opted not to contradict her too much in anticipation of an easier life. He did have one too many on occasion and subsequently found the Dutch courage to tell her what he thought but it was not always a good idea because we would all suffer for days after with deadly atmospheres juxtaposing sulking moods.

In reality, though, one could take my mother anywhere as she conducted herself with much grace. If we would metaphorically show our arse (I had been known to do the full moon when intoxicated), my mum would remind us that she could not understand the reasons why because she was so so (refined).

After a few months' tray packing and settling into the factory routine, it is vividly recalled that many a Friday afternoon I would be on tenterhooks, wondering if Mr Bird, the foreman, would ask me to work Saturday morning. Cyril Bird was a lean middle-aged amicable man, hailing from the local area, who wore a long white starched overall to befit his foreman status. At intervals throughout the day Mr Bird would drag open the heavy slide door to access the carton packing area where rude and grumpy Percy would pack the cardboard cartons with ware. His carton packing (as it was known) was undertaken at a very fast pace, I might add; which is probably the reason why his surly moods were countenanced by fellow workers. Percy was also middle-aged and sported gingery-dirty yellow hair that had been swept over to obscure the baldness. Directly beyond the strewn with straw carton packing area was the loading bay, and to the right were the stairs leading to the musty smelling basement where I would retrieve flat tray cartons which I would eventually make into boxes to load cups, saucers, soup tureens and a host of other fine bone china artefacts.

While packing away, on Friday afternoons in particular, my nerves would be shot as I sensed dark foreboding movements behind.

"Oh God, it's Mr Bird coming through and he is going to ask me to come in tomorrow," I would worryingly say to myself.

No, (breathing a sigh of relief) it was Winnie fetching another stack of ware.

Winnie Carter was approaching old age and wore an overall which often complimented a smart pleated skirt and blouse underneath. She talked about her husband, 'Gord', a lot and at break time we would mostly chatter about my Aunty Mary who Winnie knew when she was a girl. Apparently, in the 1950s, Winnie and her friend would comb the factories of Tunstall asking for work, and on one occasion they came across my Aunty Mary who presided over an office in one such factory. Winnie relayed how Mary would turn her nose up and would inform in dismissive belittling tones that there were no situations vacant. Winnie and I would then discuss the irony of it all, as in how Mary, who was one of nine and heralded from a council house on Greenbank Road, would end up marrying the guy that owned most of the pottery factories in Longton, which would later merge to become what was to be known as Royal Doulton.

Winnie would become very agitated if my radio had been turned up a decibel or two too loud. She preferred the oldies on Radio 2 but I was always tuned into Radio 1, who played all the latest pop. *My Way of Thinking*, UB40's first hit, always strikes a musical chord when epitomising this, the only reasonably long chapter in my physical career.

My little black radio got me through it, you see, and was the most important commodity. Alas, Winnie, at times, would make quips like 'are yer winneen' which I deduced was an invitation to converse. She was attached directly before me on the production line and was a 'checker', who checked the ware before it was packed; she always signed a little docket to say so. Attached to Winnie in reverse order was the order picker and I never knew who was attached to the order picker but do remember the lithographers who were all very luckily seated in a row not too far away from me (standing up jobs were the worst, you see).

Would there be a reprieve from Mr Bird any week soon, I would often ponder again and again, still rooted in anticipation on those cyclical Friday afternoons. As in, *just for once, would he not ask me to come in, thus allowing me to have that precious lie-in on a Saturday morning?*

I would hear footsteps and the sliding shut of the miserable steel slider door behind me. Soul-destroying tones would then echo the wording accompaniment like a cacophony of doom, the decibels of which harmonised my arduous factory floor existence.

"Are yer in termorrer, Kev?"

I did not want to come in, but instead submitted in an accepting, resigned to it, almost exhausted voice, "Yeah."

The subsequent eighteen months of my sentence were characterised by repetitive, soul-destroying hard work compounded by the physical actions of: item, wrap, tray, tape, load. It just went on and on and on. I felt like this was what it must have been like on the plantations all those years ago. Monotony aside, the imaginative segment of my brainacular would not submit.

Once upon a time, while wrapping a fancy-looking coffee pot and being careful to separate the lid from the base, a little spider was discovered inside the pot. Fully immersed in storybook mode it was decided to allow 'Spidey' to emigrate to Australia as that was the destination for which that particular coffee pot was destined. I had placed a little note into the pot explaining that Spidey had always dreamed of emigrating to Oz to start a new life so please could they look after him because he could well be disorientated after his long and difficult journey from England.

I remembered how my bulbous face crimsoned while my teenage boils must have simultaneously twinkled like little red cinders on a pinkly flushed tapestry when that particular order had been returned and management had viewed my little export ditty concealed inside the coffee pot.

Well, my imagination was alive, if the soul was dead, I rationalised, to counteract my inherent embarrassment.

Factory life also included the Lump Sales where one rummaged through the porcelain seconds at rock bottom prices. The sales were held in my dinner hour which would enable me to get my mum what I could within the limited time frame. This was, of course, on condition that it was not a Tuesday afternoon, which was staff chippy day, when a 'mixture' (chips and mushy peas) was on the menu. Yes, I can almost sense that potato fried in oil aroma. Imagine my horror after acquiring many pieces in the Cornpoppy design to notice those same pieces chipped and cracked in my mum's kitchen weeks later. To say it was insulting was an understatement. Cornpoppy was a sought-after design which reflected the Art Nouveau revival of the 1960s and early 70s, influenced by artists like Mucha. The image on this particular fine bone china was of a corn poppy in red and olive green, on a white, delicate, porcelain background.

I can also remember when it was my mum's birthday and she anticipated a nice piece of Wedgwood Jasper jewellery that I could also purchase at discount prices. Instead I got her one of those large drinking glasses which featured a mouse inside, with a cat climbing up the outside. Talk about pulling her face (looking miserable) when she made the discovery.

Talking of Jasperware (a type of fine-grained unglazed stoneware first developed by Josiah Wedgwood in the 1770s), towards the end of my working sentence I purchased some pieces to give to a school friend's mother who lived in North Wales. Rita was striking for her age and had moved from her native Ireland to marry a Welshman and settle in Abergele. Her eldest son and I both attended Blessed Edward Jones High School in Rhyl together. Rita was an Everton supporter, so when she came over to Stoke-on-Trent in December 1980 for the Wedgwood pieces we naturally convened at the old Victoria Ground for the First Division Stoke City vs Everton fixture. Before the game, which ended in a 2-2 draw (attendance: 15,650) I handed over some Queen's Jubilee plates in light blue and white Jasper. It came as no surprise when Rita asked if there were any plaques featuring the Pope's image instead.

"Sell them," I replied letting her know that yours truly wasn't a keen Royalist either.

To summarise my eighteen-month stretch inside Susie Cooper's, one can categorically state that it would not have been on the bucket list of things to do before one expires. The highlight of every working day was the tallying of my dockets, which took place in the office on one of those adding machines which was adjacent to my toiling area. I was on piece work. By packing more of the purple-boxed fancies my tally would be much higher because there was no need to wrap the items in paper. Mr Bird would smile when my personal tally was high, bearing in mind that my packing record was that of 7,100 pieces in one day (but on that occasion most of the orders had been fancies).

After tallying, I would sprinkle water around my packing area to quell the dust and brush up. At this time a tangible sense of relief would be sensed because the servitude would then be over – at least for another day.

Many could argue as to why anybody would work in factories like Susie Cooper if they loathed it so much. Well those who espouse that argument do not understand the working classes of that generation. It did not matter what job one did as long as one was working. In reality, it felt like being punished for over 340 days a year, if we take into consideration the customary Potters' Holiday, which was a permanent annual fixture held on the last week of June and the first week in July. The unfortunates could then get some respite from it all by holidaying in Rhyl or Towyn.

It is also recalled that cooperating, conforming and compliant serfs also had their perks, which in turn could induce fierce sibling rivalry.

"Why are there cans of Coke in the fridge for Kevin?" one family member would bemoan, since I was the only one to drink Coca Cola.

Who knows, our unknowing mother could well have been indoctrinating the next generational slave, in that there were rewards for hard work, you know.

There's nowt like the working-class ethos; an unwritten code that simultaneously imprisons and perpetuates the ideation that tray packing on the plantation was the right and proper thing to do. What's more, one was also supposed to feel a proud sense of loyalty for doing so.

The Susie Cooper factory closed in December 1980 and I was not unhappy on hearing the news we were to be made redundant. I could have sworn that, when exiting the factory gates at dusk on that last and final day, Susie's tear-stained face silhouetting the office window could be seen. I can vividly recall her pale reflection which contrasted the harsh industrial Potteries skyline – but that's another story.

Photographing Celebs at the National Football Museum

The National Football Museum in Manchester is an affordable and easily accessible day out. The museum is situated adjacent to Manchester Victoria railway station in the Cathedral Gardens area of the city.

Admission is free and there is also an under-fives children's play area called the 'Discovery Zone'. In fact, the museum is an Aladdin's cave for kids of all ages, featuring numerous interactive pursuits including football plus simulation.

To get to the museum from Manchester Piccadilly railway station, it is better to jump on the free shuttle to Manchester Victoria or get the Metro/ Tram at Piccadilly (direction Bury). The fare is nominal. The museum is also well within walking distance from Piccadilly.

On entering the building, look to the right-hand side for the interior cable car. This novel contraption can elevate the less mobile to all the museum tiers (including the bar and restaurant on the upper floors).

This odd-shaped former Urbis building (now the museum) is shaped like a short staircase with four levels housing the exhibits. This very modern piece of architecture seems almost at odds married to a display of historical footballing nostalgia; being mindful that the museum had formerly been located at Preston North End's Deepdale Stadium until 2009.

I have a special bond with the museum because it was where I managed to obtain my cherished photograph of the major celeb, Victoria Beckham.

Yes, I took the snap on the ground floor, near to the restaurant.

You'd never guess it was a photograph of a cardboard cut-out.

Just a Selection of 'Care' Home Incidents

Log of incidents

All through 2015, up to my mother's CHC assessment in November, there were reports of her falling out of bed, which are supported by images taken by me, her son. There were also complaints both in 2015 and 2016 of my mother having dirty fingernails. This proud, dignified woman was also at the end of her life.

April 18th 2016, at 13.05 my mother was again in a precarious position at the edge of the bed. Her sporadic behaviour had rendered her in great danger of falling out. It was only when I intervened that she was repositioned by care workers.

April 23rd 2016, (Saturday) at 12.45 my mum's appearance was unkempt and her nightdress was open to reveal her breast area. My mother's arms were also not covered, cognisant that I had already informed the manager of the care home that due to her frailty she should wear a long-sleeved nightdress. My mother appeared thirsty as she continually licked her lips and was also in a dangerous position where her head was positioned to the side as if she could struggle to breathe. My mum's care plan stated that she must be visited by a care worker every fifteen minutes. What's more, it had been marked in the book that she had been visited at 12.45. Then again, I was there at 12.45 and no care worker visited. Subsequently, there was no visit, at 13.00 or 13.15. A care worker appeared at 13.30 and only then repositioned her (due to her precarious position) because I was present.

It is believed there is an instrument that other homes use to verify that the patient has been checked. I requested this instrument should be used at the care home but could not request this to the home directly as the relationship with the care home in question had broken down.

July 2nd 2016, at approximately 11.00, I was distressed to see my mother's pyjama top around her neck, which could have hampered her breathing. Her breast area was exposed again. The blue mattress she was lying on appeared dirty where the undercover was pulled up under my mum to expose the mattress which also would render my mother extremely uncomfortable. One of the care workers (a guy in his 40s) later stated that if I was not happy with my mum's care I should move her, as in that is what he would do if it was his mother. I replied that any move could kill my mother. The care worker then disclosed that he had checked her at 10.30 and she had been checked again at 10.45 and nothing untoward was reported. He also clearly stated that within fifteen minutes my mother can wriggle to such an extent she can render herself into the position which I witnessed at 11.00. This suggests that my mum was in need of one-on-one care as a priority.

July 24th 2016, I received a phone call to inform me that a stranger had entered my mother's room and put a mattress over her and pulled the pump out of her support bed. It is therefore unknown if other strangers (or the same one) had previously entered her room, taking into consideration the door to her room had been open since early 2015. The matter was reported to East Cheshire Local Authority.

August 16th 2016, I visited the home on this date to find my mother lying on her bed in just her pads. This was humiliating and was witnessed by another person. We both came to the conclusion that the alarm mat positioned by the care home to detect strangers entering my mum's room was not foolproof as you can easily step over it.

October 1st 2016, at 10.00, when I visited my mother she was being fed breakfast. She was not wearing long sleeves on her nightdress even though I had repeatedly requested she be dressed in long sleeves because of her frailty. Besides, the temperature had dropped to 10 degrees outside. After being fed, my mother was left lying flat on her back which appeared like the bed was set in a wrong, disagreeable-looking (some would say dangerous) position and when I pointed out my concern to one of the two new young care workers, one care worker said that was the bed position she had been told to leave my mother in. I went to find a more experienced care worker who stated that the bed was in the wrong position and repositioned it. I had to request that the more experienced care worker show the new care worker what position my mum and the bed should be left in. This is basic care and it is not for a relative to point out how his mother should be positioned. The manager was on duty at the time and was ignorant of the situation. It makes one wonder what would have ensued if I had not visited that day.

October 20th 2016, I received a telephone call from the nurse at the home (19.20). He informed me that my mother had been found with a deep black bruise on her hand measuring 8cm by 4cm. He said that he had checked with the manager if my mother had had any bloods done which could have caused the bruising but was assured that no bloods or anything like had been undertaken. I advised that the nurse call in the doctor, who visited the care home the very next day. I also informed a representative of the CQC (Care Quality Commission) and an agent from the social care team in Stoke-on-Trent via email to register the incident. As you can imagine, I was very upset and worried, considering everything that had gone on previously (a safeguarding investigation by Cheshire East Council regarding my mother's care had supposedly just been undertaken).

October 21st 2016, I visited the care home on this day and took a photograph of my mother's bruised hand. Last time I visited it was reported that my mother's bed was positioned flat which was the wrong setting to safeguard her health. The bed was in exactly the same, wrong position seen previously, which rendered my mother flat on her back again. There appeared to be more agency staff on duty than usual and when I pointed the bed position out to an agency worker she replied that she had not been shown how to position the bed. Another care worker also mentioned that 'all the staff were leaving'.

After a lengthy Ombudsman investigation which concluded in December 2017, one council was exonerated, and the other was found to have caused me an injustice (the Ombudsman found against them). Therefore, the council found blameworthy (in parts don't forget) were told to complete care plans in future, oh and I nearly forgot, they were ordered to apologise to me and award me £150 in compensation.

Rebranding our Stadia:
A Bitter Pill to Swallow

The modern era of football advertisement has not only taken the football shirt off our backs (the club name on the shirt is now secondary to the sponsor) we have seen our historic and original stadia name changed. The reason given for the name changes at many stadiums over the years is that revenue from sponsorship would be used to buy players or to save the club from going into administration. Makes one wonder then how players were bought in years gone by, doesn't it? What is worse, we never hear any criticism from those who front football in England and Wales regarding the pillaging and name ruination of our clubs by the multi-national. We saw St James' Park, home of Newcastle United, known as the Sports Direct Arena for a short time. Then we had poor old Coventry City suffering the Highfield Road/Ricoh Arena shambles and traditional West Ham United enduring the humiliation of trying to adjust to the 'Wide Track Olympic Park'. Not to mention Manchester City. Maine Road was a treat. What is their football ground now called? Yes, the Etihad. And Arsenal, the gloss was taken off the fashionable Highbury when it changed to the Emirates wasn't it? Apparently, it was on the cards in 2017 that the governing families of the United Arab Emirates, who control the Emirates and Etihad airlines, might hold talks regarding possibly merging the two. It gets worse, doesn't it?

Bolton Wanderers supporters probably drew the short straw with the Reebok Stadium. The setting gives the mercantile game away; the ground is based at Middlebrook Retail Park. It can be said therefore that the absurdity of naming our stadiums after commercial enterprises contradicts itself in the basest of fashions; in 2009, Reebok announced plans to pull out of the town (which had its headquarters at the Reebok Stadium) and to consider proposals to end its 116-year history in Bolton. Where does that leave the fans – with an empty commercial shell once known as their football ground? Currently in 2018, it is unclear if Bolton's ground is called the Macron Stadium or the University of Bolton Stadium.

Is it not high time to return to the original names of our football grounds? Some deem that Stoke City were lucky. Changing the name of the Victoria Ground to the Britannia Stadium still had historical and cultural resonance. In spite of this, it would go from bad to worse for long-established Stoke City supporters, the ground has now been named after a gambling company (the bet365 Stadium). What next bet365 FC? What was insulting for Stoke fans is that the name change was announced at exactly the same time ground capacity was announced to be increased (to over 30,000) in an attempt to soften the blow.

Talking of the Wiganesque, Wigan Athletic, when in the Premier League, may have been instrumental in the trend of repeatedly changing the names of our arenas. First the JJB stadium, now the DW Stadium, whatever next; KitKat Crescent? Joking aside, from 2005–2010 York City's Bootham Crescent was known just as that.

Another incongruity is naming football clubs after the owners or directors. Reading and Oxford United are prime examples of vanity and egos out of control. Sir John Robert Madejski is no longer associated with the Madejski Stadium (formerly known as Elm Park) but the name remains the same. Reading is now 90.29% owned by Renhe Sports Management Co Ltd (which is owned 100% by Mr Yongge Dai), confusing isn't it? In reference to Oxford United; Firoz Kassam has departed from the club but refused to sell it on, so the Kassam Stadium (the name of the ground) still remains.

Then we had Vincent Tan, owner of Cardiff City, going one step further by changing the clubs home strip from blue to red. Although the decision was reversed after fan pressure. How dare he?

Many football fans today feel removed from the game and it can be said that it's dangerous to tamper with the nucleus or soul of the club (the grounds) for commercial gain; but the powers that be do so anyway. This is in turn engendering many to feel that fan ownership of clubs is being taken away from supporters by the massive conglomerates. Ordinary people don't have much to call their own, but with a football club they have a common interest where they pay monies into a club to sustain that interest. They are collectively known as football supporters.

Freakos

Chicos, a nightclub in Hanley, used to be open on Tuesday and Friday evenings for popular dance and on Saturday evenings, in the late 1970s and very early 1980s, for the New Romantics. After 1982, Saturday evening was designated for students or the alternatives. My face can still cringe with embarrassment when recalling one Saturday night when I dyed my hair blue and freaked out at Freakos, as we later called it. I was well smashed.

The clientele on a Saturday evening could sometimes appear androgynous with their way-out clothes and hairstyles. We could also have troops of nasty drunken apes marauding the streets of Hanley in those days and anyone with a varied appearance, heaven help them. I reckon those New Romantic types must have drawn up in a taxi to Charles Street and made a quick dash for Chicos door before an eagle-eyed lookout in Ape Troop spotted them.

Back in the 1980s, one's whole life revolved around meeting that special person on a Friday or a Saturday night, wearing your new togs, of course. For some, that special person never arrived. On the contrary, many would run for the hills when they saw yours truly roll in blotto.

If out on a Friday evening, the Olde French Horn was frequented first for a few liveners; the Frenchie, as we called it, was the original inn place to be. *Take Me I'm Yours*, Squeeze and *World In My Eyes*, Depeche Mode, could be blaring out from the jukebox put on by none other than me, who fancied himself as the true connoisseur of all good things music. I would always try and boss the tunes. We would then walk around to Chicos before eleven, where we could meet the odd coarse braggart along the way, one of which once declared, because I was wearing sunglasses, "Look, he is wearing sunglasses at night."

347

There could be seen many a Backward Barry up Anley duck.

If I was sober enough and in the club early, there would be time for a serious strut to hits like *Pump Up The Jam*, Technotronic. On the other hand, the saying at Chicos, when getting late in the evening was, "Ten to two grab a screw".

On one Tuesday evening I was so deleteriously drunk I was frogmarched out of the nightclub after having a scuffle. I could never take me ale, you know.

On another occasion, I foolishly tried a strange drug and at first it was amusing turning into professor Kev, analysing the strange cavorting human species involved in the bizarre mating ritual. However, it was short-lived. All of a sudden, and figuratively speaking, of course, the ceiling collapsed and I felt quite disturbed. I rushed out of Chicos with my coat over my head so no one could see my, by now, very peculiar looking boat-race. I was so paranoid I did not even bother to purchase my customary pudding, chips and peas from the chip van parked nearby.

The year was 1989.

Note: Chicos was badly damaged by fire in 2003, having closed its doors for the last time just three weeks before.

The Outcast

The moral question that needs to be asked immediately is how our so-called Christian church/government officials can address the sad, modern-day social outrage regarding those isolated. What about compulsory checks by wellbeing teams for those over sixty-five? The teams could offer those living alone contact details of others suffering alone. If the checks were obligatory, there would be no embarrassment for the lonely person/s visited.

As families and friends gather as part of everyday routine, we should spare a thought for the lonely and estranged. For those in our community who have nobody, life can be painful and distressing, resulting in some falling into deep despair.

In 2018, the number of those living solo in Britain has more than doubled in comparison to the early 1970s. Consequently, those living isolationary lives sees them spending much more per year on household bills in comparison to their coupled counterparts.

There is also strong empirical evidence regarding the link between isolation and ill-health. The most vulnerable groups are the elderly, the disabled, single parents, the bereaved and those divorced or separated. The bad news for those living alone is that they are more likely to die prematurely; they have more chance of suffering heart disease, tuberculosis, accidents, mental health difficulties and are more likely to commit suicide.

It's unknown why some people find themselves excluded and yes, a small percentage of human beings do prefer to live that way. Some get used to the state of solitariness as a way of life having experienced 'cluster living' and as a result finding the group scenario unsettling.

On the contrary, some do not always make a conscious choice to become isolated, but find themselves entombed in solitude for long periods by chance or circumstance.

When becoming an outcast for long periods, some can lose their power of speech. What is not widely understood is that talking and conversation in general is an acquired art form and one has to continually practice to stay fluent. When those who spend too much time alone stop practicing dialogue they can and do lose that power of communication.

Keeping in mind, of course, that in a gaol of one's own making there is no release date; one just hopes and prays for a pardon. But what happens to the inner spirit when in confinement? One does not have to consult the Socratic school of spiritual philosophy to understand that our spirit is a sense or definition of who we are and when we are starved of human companionship that essence dies. The reason for this is because the inner spirit needs other positive spirits in order to survive. In effect, our spirit 'bounces off' another person's spirit in order to feed back to ourselves who we are as human beings and how we fit into the generic scheme of things. It can be safely deduced that it is through other people that we make sense of our own lives.

Those who are socially privileged in our society should try to imagine what they would do if everybody they knew suddenly disappeared. They would not just be shell-shocked, they would lose their sense of identity, place in the world, significance, and ultimately they would be lost.

There are people in our communities who have lost everything and everybody and have been trapped in this limbo, sometimes for years.

The point also has to be made that, although our inner spirit seeks out other kindred spirits to enable healthy relationships and a sense of wellbeing, poor relationships are due to a corruption of the fusing spirits where we should look to get out of such negative relationships as soon as possible. People can induce stress on one another to such an extent that it would have a negative impact on the value of each other's lives, that is why it is all-important to strike the right balance with social relationships; the emphasis being on quality not quantity – we are a group-orientated species.

Unquestionably, it is nice to have one's own space to collect one's thoughts and to be viewed as the strong, silent independent type in not being reliant on others. Especially when you consider that hard men have been known to break down and sob when faced with the notion of being alone.

But the big question is why does seclusion become a way of life for some? And what's more, what enables that strange paradox where some find a painful comfort in being totally segregated because they are so accustomed to solitude?

In this instance, the practicalities of habitual social interaction has been turned upside down where instead of feeling uneasy when consistently isolated they feel relaxed. Conflictingly, when intermittently interacting with others the loner feels nervous and unsettled, and so this pattern becomes impressed.

It is also believed that there are three degrees or thresholds of isolation. Firstly, there is the concept of 'solitary', where one is alone most of the time, then there is the state of 'semi-solitary' (where some could work full-time but spend the intervening leisure time alone) and last but not least we have 'super solitary' where one passes every waking hour unaccompanied. It is thought the three degrees of solitude are fluid, as in people can continually move into and out of all three states of remoteness.

Substance abuse can keep one isolated too. Without even being aware of it many of us could be engaging in an intense one-on-one relationship with our escape medicine of choice; to soothe the dull ache of spaced-out nothingness.

In summary, many lonely and segregated people learn to live cyber-lives and communicate mainly through technological apparatus like the Internet. Still, it should be remembered that this substitute relationship is ultimately occurring with a machine, not a person.

There's No Fool Like an Old Fool

Visiting the British Museum in London recently, where the Ancient British 'Lindow Man' was exhibited, enables other self-discussions to surface. Thought to be from the mid-1st century AD, this aged discovery was excavated in Cheshire, England, in 1984, when workmen were cutting peat at Lindow Moss bog.

Scientific research has allowed us to learn more about this person (his health, his appearance and how he might have died) than any other prehistoric body found in Britain. The conditions in the peat bog meant that the man's skin, hair and many of his internal organs are well preserved. Radiocarbon dating shows that he died between 2BC and AD119. He was about twenty-five years of age, around 168cm tall and weighed 60–65kg.

Several Prehistoric bog bodies have been discovered all over Europe and although there are numerous theories circulating regarding their lives and subsequent violent deaths, the simple answer is that they were more than likely all clan leaders. Whereas, as another invading tribe took control of an area, the clan leader was removed and buried in a remote spot.

We might not all appear well-preserved after 2,000 years in the bog, but age is an odd conundrum, and today, as we all grow older, what have we learnt?

I was on a bus, on the way back from the museum, close to Tavistock Place in Central London, when I noted an older woman leaving the bus. As she did so, she kind of leaned against a younger, but middle-aged gentleman for support. The gentlemen in question was obviously not the genteel or compassionate type, because he shrugged her off and uttered a rude comment at the same time. I observed that the older woman was quite taken aback and her aging plumage visibly ruffled. I watched her step off the bus at the junction of Euston Road, where she noticeably quickened her step. Therefore, had the impolite and uncompassionate stranger initiated a survival mechanism in the older woman and actually helped her, as in had he enabled the penny to drop that she could not always rely on others, and many would not wish to be burdened with her?

Staying with real-life puzzles that can often be witnessed on public transport, we also have the expression 'invisibles'. This referent apparently applies to unnoticed older people on a bus or train. How odd for people to be subconsciously classed as bland, uniform and invisible to the human eye because of age. This fast, take your money as quickly as possible, culture does not help matters. Many a time one can see older people struggling to keep up with the pace where they can fumble when paying their fare or retrieving tickets on public transport; usually to the dismay of the queue forming behind. Wouldn't it be refreshing if a flummoxed older person at the front of the queue just turned around and stuck up the V sign.

From a personal perspective, on hitting my thirties, I began to understand older people. My younger thinking believed my twenties would last indefinitely and those in their forties were old. Around the thirty mark, I stopped watching current popular culture TV shows like *Top of the Pops* featuring the latest hits. Perhaps it was a sign I was coming of age in that my reproductive peak had well, peaked, and I did not need to participate in the mating dance ritual any more. Of mind that in one's forties and fifties, twenty, thirty, or even forty years ago does not seem a long time, but in one's twenties it seemed like an eternity.

As we age, we see our bodies (including face and frame) change very slowly for the worse, where one can struggle to upload and post a recent presentable image (that does not make you look old) online. Then, around the sixty mark, the indelible shadow sets in which you can do nothing about. Old age has caught up with you but you can soften the blow by kidding yourself that some people are into oldies. There's no fool like an old fool.

At this crossroads you can either curl up and die or get older; you only have two choices (there is the option of investing in expensive creams or plastic surgery; but it will all head south in the end). Getting older can mean joining the other water dinosaurs at your local swimming baths, thus wading through the pool because you are too old to swim. You can also use the word 'youngsters' a lot and repeat the phrase 'when I was your age' over and over.

Or better still, you can just be thankful that at this intersection in your life you do not have to worry about the things you used to worry about.

You haven't got the time.

Out of the Ordinary in Blackpool

When growing up it was always one or the other at holiday time: Rhyl or Blackpool, that is. This does not mean that it was any less exciting; as a child one prepared to enter another universe when holiday time came around.

One can argue that Blackpool still has the allure of the English kind which dates back to the mid-19th century when the 'working classes' first began to visit. Little has changed; we still have rain, amusement arcades, shows (curiosities), pubs, gift shops, a promenade, funfairs, candy floss/ toffee apples, rock, seagulls, donkey rides and fish & chips.

And the more recent resort gimmick like those cringey 'Kiss me Quick' hats.

No, we do not have weather like the continental climes, but in stating the obvious, stormy days in Blackpool can still be as entertaining, especially when the Irish Sea turns on the rough charm. Then we have that strange occurrence where the sea air can virtually 'knock you out' (it has been known for some people to sleep for twelve hours uninterrupted after spending time out and about in Blackpool).

The more cultured and worldly travelled among us should not turn their noses up at Blackpool. The town in the North West can teach us a thing or two about what it is to be English.

Blackpool can educate us as to what it means to be one of the majority classes and how innocently thrilling it is to bunk down in a guest house, B&B, chalet or even a caravan and to wake up to that 'full English' breakfast the following morning by the sea.

Simple holidays on the British coast can help the independent observer comprehend how human beings find succour in everything familiarly modest.

Some would also declare, in criticism, that Blackpool is marred by drunken revelry and is best avoided by the more discerning after dark. Others would go one further and say that the 'naked carousing' practiced in the early hours borders on anarchy.

This may well be the case.

We can also bear witness to those inebriated groups of males/females all attired in the same party outfits, participating in some inane mating ritual or display – what is that all about?

The answer is not out of the ordinary; it is about people being people.

And that is what Blackpool is about: ordinary people.

The Second Dimension

I have seen those lost ashen faces on display at the local bookies (bookmakers). Paled, demeaned from losing their benefits, their wages, their mortgage payments or even something more substantial. Those wan-troubled expressions can often be seen affixed to roulette machines otherwise known as fixed-odds betting terminals. What's the answer – ban these machines?

A gambling compulsion is an addictive condition like any other addiction; it destroys lives in just the same manner. While lucky in not suffering from this particular malady myself (I like a flutter but know my limits), others are not so lucky. I can recall when I got five numbers on the National Lottery. Although only receiving £1,082 in winnings, seven hundred and seventy-seven people got five numbers that week (777). Yes, the three sevens were up.

Talking of lucky combinations, during my first visit to Uttoxeter racecourse a few years back, a fortuitous second dimension combination arose. When I chose my four horses for a £5 accumulator, I did so fully aware that the last train home was 9pm. So, after the first horse went down, I had to accumulate again. As a result, I did not include Sheriff Hutton, who would be competing in the last race. If I had added Sheriff Hutton to make a four-horse accumulation and stayed for the last race, I would have missed the last train home. Consequently, I opted for a three-horse accumulator instead.

My first horse, Lord Alfred, strolled home at around 6/1, my second, Galaxia, then romped home at 12/1, so it all hinged on Harry Potter, priced at 5/1. Waiting with baited breath at the finishing post, Harry Potter struggled around the course and neared the back-marker for most of the time. It was all change in the final furlong when he began to make strong ground. I purred in polite glee (like the cat that got the cream) as Harry Potter pipped the leading horse at the post. All my three horses had won.

Feeling blessed at my good fortune, the counter assistant quipped, "1976." This signified that I had won £24 off £2,000. Yes, I felt like the High Sheriff of Staffordshire as I strode toward the railway station to catch the last train home. Why wouldn't I? There was a big bulging wad of notes bursting out of my back pocket.

On the station platform, I could hear the final race commence on loudspeaker (of which I couldn't attend for fear of missing the last train home) and of course, my fourth chosen horse (but not betted on), Sheriff Hutton, won. If there had been a later train, I would have pocketed around £12,000.

Mulling it over on the train, it was conjectured that if I had indeed backed four horses instead of three as intended, would I have missed the last train home to watch the last race (where Sheriff Hutton would be competing) with my three horses already in the bag, of mind that I would have had to book an expensive taxi home if Sheriff Hutton had lost. Furthermore, if Sheriff Hutton had lost, I would have also lost the accrued £1,976 and come away with nothing. Don't forget, my £1,976 would now have been riding on Sheriff Hutton.

At this place and time, that second dimension quandary entered the arena.

Was it therefore the right decision to have accumulated just the three horses and come away with £1,976? And most importantly, if I had accumulated four horses, how would the final race have unfolded? In that, if I had attended the fourth race in person, could the course of events have changed due to my physical presence at the race and as a result Sheriff Hutton lost? For example, what if a colour I was wearing had put the horse off? Or might some kind of behind the scenes activity have occurred, in mind that a lucky punter (me) would be walking out of the racecourse with £12,000?

It was concluded that I was very fortunate for the monies secured, thank you very much.

By my reckoning, £1,976 in the hand is worth more than £12,000 in the bush.

Wiping the Slate Clean

It seems a travesty that those who have previously been trapped in the dark abyss of addiction and petty criminality cannot move on from their 'crimes'.

The Criminal Records Bureau (CRB) and the Independent Safeguarding Authority (ISA) have recently merged into the Disclosure and Barring Service (DBS) but that has not altered the policy of criminal records being 'spent'.

One person with addiction problems and currently in recovery who, while immersed in addiction, accrued convictions for petty shoplifting, has since requested the DBS check so they could begin to volunteer within the social sphere.

On being non-textbook, the volunteer could possibly influence others that are considering immersing themselves into a life of addiction and petty crime, as in they can pass on their lived knowledge to current would-be addicts and offenders.

This ex-offender who is wishing to be rehabilitated and move back into mainstream society is systematically held back. On the resulting DBS certificate (which was as long as their arm) it was noted the details of shoplifting convictions dating back to the 1970s.

Absurd, isn't it?

It is the essence of humanitarian decency to forgive and allow someone to shed that old skin and move forward.

Harsh government measures do not facilitate those (who have not offended against children) to evolve from their past but to remain locked into it.

It's time that non-serious offences were wiped clean after five years.

We can Call our Country England

The word England has become so rare in everyday vernacular it is as though many are afraid to use it. That word, dare I say it, England, has all but been expelled from our native tongue; firstly by Great Britain (which includes the Kingdoms of England, Scotland and the principality of Wales) and secondly by that annoying UK (which stands for the United Kingdom of Great Britain and Northern Ireland).

The once popular words Great Britain, British, and the British Isles are also becoming suffocated by the phrase 'UK', perhaps because of overuse by the established media. Then, of course, the phrase is duly parroted by the masses.

Consequently, should our official language not be known as English but UKish?

I don't know about anybody else but that piercing utterance 'UK', emphasising the sound 'Kay', goes through one more than licking a chalky blackboard – especially when emanating from that so-called high-bred superficial London RP twang (with loads of ifs and bots in between). It makes one muse as to how our controllers will refer to the 'UK' if Scotland votes for its own independence. Will the 'UK' be known as: 'The UK minus Scotland' or 'The UK including Wales and Six Little Counties of Ireland'?

It is so ludicrous you would imagine the contradictory trappings of the 'UK' to be a work of fiction. The facts are that there is a simple solution to our confusing landmass piece of faction.

We can call our country England.

Demonstrations at Wedgwood for the Select Few

Costing £7.50 in 2015 (£5 concessions) the Wedgwood Museum in Barlaston can be difficult to locate because of the lack of appropriate signposting. The car parking area was also confusing when visited in 2015. It is hoped that these teething problems are now resolved as the complex begins to take shape in light of the recent £34m 'World of Wedgwood' redevelopment.

The factory tour has been custom-built and is thought to be equipped with nineteen stations and viewing platforms to observe the pottery (or potbank) production lines. There is also a section open to the public where local craftsmen and women give demonstrations. Apparently embroidering the Jasperware with the beautiful leaf design is still undertaken by the same moulding technique as was used in the eighteen hundreds. In the same area you can throw a pot yourself and have it sent on to your home address.

I had previously visited the museum itself in 2012 and remember that one could have their photo taken by the virtual portrait interactive machine that casts your image into a Jasper frame.

My personal favourites inside the museum are the First Day's Vase of 1769 (in July, 2017 the vase was saved from being exported to the USA after £482,500 was raised to keep it at the museum) and the Jasper-emblazoned perambulator dated 1963. Adjacent to the museum entrance is the free tea sampling area called the Wedgwood Tea Emporium, which is in turn annexed to the beautiful Wedgwood Tea Room. Sandwiches and tea at the rooms are expensive, as is the confectionery in the Dining Hall (the restaurant across the way). To order a pot of tea for £2 at the Dining Hall is reasonable, bearing in mind you can ask for an extra cup and share the brew.

The staff at the World of Wedgwood are approachable, informative and professional. In saying that one employee in the Wedgwood Tea Emporium appeared rather perplexed when I enquired as to whether the teas to sample bore any relation to Josiah. As in, did he sip any of them from one of his cups while relaxing in the drawing room. It's good for the visitor to identify directly with our Master Potter Josiah Wedgwood.

On the same theme (cups and tea) during my first visit in 2012, a kind lady working in the restaurant said I could take the 'Wild Strawberry' patterned bone china beaker, in which I had just drunk my tea, home with me. I left a £1 tip as a thank you. I still have the mug today which is currently the only vessel I will drink my tea and coffee from.

The 'Wild Strawberry' design, still featuring on displayed fine bone china around the complex, took me back to when I worked for the company in the years 1979–80. The factory was called Susie Cooper, on Newcastle Street in Burslem, which was part of the Wedgwood Group. Yours truly was a tray packer (I still do demonstrations today for the select few which features repetitive hand and arm flailing to express how hard I worked in pulling the paper from a roll to pack the ware in trays). As well as the boxed Jasper, I packed the Wild Strawberry and other patterned pieces for export ('Cornpoppy' and 'Glen Mist' were other beautiful designs, as detailed in the article 'Are You Winnie?').

Have You Been, Walter?

Newsnight on BBC2 (September 19th 2012) was cause for a titter or two. Liberal Democrat Business Secretary, Vince Cable, being quizzed by Jeremy Paxman regarding his party's pre-election promises of no increase in student tuition fees, saw him calling the Deputy Prime Minister Nick Clegg, Nick Pledge instead.

It unfolded in the programme item that pledges made by twister Nick Clegg not to increase student fees were a mistake. In his defence, sycophant Clegg had apologised via a sort of politico-surreal broadcast that the Lib Dems had "promised things his party could not deliver". It was almost a new twist on reneging what politicians promise before an election and what they actually dispense.

Clegg though, reminded more of Nellie Pledge (Hylda Baker) and Cable, Walter Tattershall (played by Edward Malin) in the dated comedy show *Nearest and Dearest*. There was even a physical comparison between Walter and Vince, where Cable exuberated that docile 'Walter look' specially for Newsnight viewers. Cable got his lines crossed and looked visibly shaken throughout the broadcast, as he mumbled his way around the fact of whether he knew his party could not/would not keep student fees to a minimum. In fact, when Cable did call Clegg 'Pledge' the audience (now used to this pair of hilarious bumbling nitwits) half-expected the Deputy Prime Minister to enter the stage delivering the classic line: "Have you been, Walter?"

Talk about typecasting. In *Nearest and Dearest*, which ran from 1968 – 1973, Walter, the ever-silent elderly husband of Lily, spent most of his time doddering to and from the toilet, or sitting extremely quietly in the Pledges' front room drinking tea. Overall though, the gist of the *Nearest and Dearest* script saw

Nellie and Eli Pledge inherit a pickle factory in the north of England which was collapsing forthwith. The company was not failing because of business acumen deficiencies, but because they had inherited a workforce that was well over retirement age. No doubt in line with the narrow and small-minded Cable and Clegg Remain rationale, the dissolving pickle empire must have all been down to Brexit.

Pompeii 2011: You Couldn't See Me for Dust

It is hard to be objective and not to generalise in today's opinionated society, but the three-day break in Naples on a budget (with the sole objective of visiting Pompeii and Vesuvius) did not come anywhere near the standards set by Rome, Venice and Florence, already visited.

The flight to Naples from Liverpool was reasonably priced and it took all but three hours. The hotel was chosen because of its central location (Piazza Garibaldi) being adjacent to the main railway station in Naples (Stazione de Napoli Centrale), of mind that I would need the station for visits to Pompeii. Naples city centre was a nightmare. To negotiate the busy main roads even on a zebra crossing was a struggle in itself. It was a game of cat and mouse one soon deduced; the vehicle owners were the cats and you were the mouse crossing at your own peril to the 'peep peeps' of irate Neapolitans on their way to God knows where. Maybe one should afford some understanding, in that the berserk motorists were more than likely in a rush to sign the Treaty of Versailles.

Sarcasm aside, it really was nerve-wracking.

The hotel was a disappointment as the rooms were basic and a little tacky, and there was no lift. It was a relief, therefore, to be on the second floor, although others were not as fortunate and made their feelings known when lugging heavy cases up flights of stairs. The whole square was like a huge bombsite and was being completely restructured, making the view from the terrace hardly pleasurable. Like the Brits with the stiff upper lip, one is supposed to just get on with it and draw comfort from the fact that from the hotel it was only a two-minute walk to the railway station, enabling the visitor to do one as often as possible.

The first day was spent acclimatising to the bedlam of Naples, which was ignorant, dirty, chaotic, unassuming and, last but not least, a little dodgy. Some of the day was spent people watching, taking into consideration that some Italian 'stunners' contrasted the dull dereliction. McDonald's was then visited for lunch, which is no cheap option by the way. Yes, when in doubt a Big Mac meal is a viable option. One was brave enough to sample the savoury Italian pastries in abundance at a later date, after having 'a good look at them first'. The internet cafés, by the way, in the city centre, reminded of squalid death traps where users produced their own toxic cloud of smoke puffing on cigarettes. As the first day drew to a close one then took a couple of slugs of liquor to calm the Neapolitan shock and got out of the way in going to bed (which was comfy at least). It was exhausting in the 28-degree heat.

The very next day, breakfast at the hotel was definitely not what mamma used to make. Cardboard bread and cornflakes with slices of cheap ham and cheese washed down with lukewarm coffee just about summed it up. On making the way to Napoli railway station to go to Pompeii one soon learnt to sort of bluff it and stride across the busy main roads like the Neapolitans do. The ignorance of staff at the railway station knew no bounds when I asked for train tickets to Pompeii. When the information desk was eventually located one felt brave enough to inform the member of staff attending (and whoever else was listening) just what was thought of these rude people.

When it was discovered that one train line to Pompeii was closed because of a strike, it reaffirmed the reasons why it was chosen to stay in Naples and not Pompeii; not just because it was less expensive than commuting to swanky Sorrento, one had to get back to the airport and Naples was only a fifteen-minute bus ride to get 'outa here'. After a polite member of the public explained how I could get to Pompeii on the Circumvesuviana line, one thanked their lucky stars; civility had been excavated amongst the throngs of swarming Italian humanity.

Taking the overcrowded train (or overground metro) from Naples to Pompeii Scava (there are two Pompeii stops) on the Sorrento-bound train, took on average forty minutes. The famous sleeping monster, the Volcano Vesuvius, can be seen at many intervals en route. At the site it cost around eleven euro for the admission fee. However, if you were over sixty-five or under eighteen you could access the location for free if producing a photocopy of your passport. The short walk to the site featured stalls selling fresh orange and lemon juice at a reasonable two euro and the souvenir shops would barter down to at least half of the marked price. Yes, the locals were helpful and civilised, unlike their Neapolitan counterparts.

I then made my way to the human plaster casts. It was down to basic morbid fascination as to how the famous archaeologist Giuseppe Fiorelli realised in the 1840s that where there were mounds of ash in Pompeii, a corpse had lain under it and decomposed over hundreds of years. The ingenious Fiorelli then poured plaster of Paris into the cavity and the ash was then removed, resulting in a replica of a person at the terrifying point of death. Death resulted no doubt from the pyroclastic surge of white hot gas and ash that poured from Vesuvius in AD79 (The Museo Archeologico Nazionale in Naples stores film on this subject matter).

There were other points of interest to be seen on the large site, like the House of Faun and the dancing Satyr and, up to October 12th, Pompeii can also be visited at night, when it's all lit up.

It must be remembered that Herculaneum is an interesting site to visit but does not possess the same pizzazz as Pompeii.

On the final day it was thought that it would be nice to visit the coast (at the hotel earlier a Paschal had stated with a straight face that he would only charge me fifty euro to take me to the bay of Naples which was only a short car ride away). He also suggested in broken English that a visit to Castellammare di Stabia on the coast, some five stops after Pompeii, was only a short walk to the shoreline. It was at this point in Castellammare, and quite by accident, that it was noticed that the perspective on Mount Vesuvius (a somma-stratovolcano) as seen from this locale had changed dramatically.

Vesuvius was not just a volcano amidst the landmass of Naples; Vesuvius was Naples itself.

The next day was home time and one left the hotel an hour early to catch the bus to the airport for the flight home, just in case.

And no, Vesuvius was not erupting again; you just couldn't see me for dust.

Big Britain

They say what the US do today we do tomorrow and as far as obesity is concerned, Britain has followed suit and is now the world's fourth fattest country. One is classed as obese if the Body Mass Index (BMI) is above thirty.

Not just a drain on the health service; the mental health problems associated with being overweight cannot be quantified. One fully understands comfort eating. The need to satiate and to fill emotional wounds with food is a well-known partiality for many. To others, eating is top of their agenda, it can be a treat and it can be a reward, but most of all it can be something to look forward to. But; what does one do when eating spirals out of control? It is easier said than done to just cut down on one's intake; to some, food is their addiction and almost their very being.

The multinational supermarket must take some of the blame for the obesity epidemic. The majority of foodstuff products are packed with either salts, sugars, saturated fats or all three. These products are projected with glossy advertisement and misleading 'good for you' guides. What can be hidden is the fact that even fresh orange juice, if concentrated, is packed with sugar, cheese is packed with fat, meats are injected with God knows what and most 'healthy cereals' are loaded with sugar and salt. What's more, nearly every food bought seems to have some carbohydrate association. Yes, education, education, education is what's needed, but where do we start?

It is recognised that it is difficult nurturing children and it is often convenient to give them 'a burger', 'a sausage roll', 'chicken nuggets' or a few sweets, especially when outdoors. Some nutritionists argue that such is the health detrimental content contained in this sort of fast-food diet that it can cause the child to become hyperactive and difficult to control. A sit down nutritional meal can induce calm and better behaviour in many children.

Bowel cancer is also associated with poor nourishment. This can someway be attributed to additives such as preservatives in food products to prolong the shelf life. Last, but not least, being overweight is not aesthetically pleasing in any way shape or form, whatever the 'pleasantly plump brigade' propagate. Being overweight demonstrates lack of control, sloppiness, laziness and even gluttony.

Did you know that the real opium of the masses, white sugar, is physically addictive and has the same properties as other drugs. Moreover, 'cold turkey', cravings, depression, fatigue, mood swings, and headaches can be attributed to sugar. Excessive sugar consumption is also believed to be involved in many common physical health problems including hypoglycaemia, heart disease, high cholesterol, obesity, indigestion, myopia, seborrheic dermatitis, gout, hyperactivity and diabetes. The cold reality being; you could wind up having a leg amputated. Then there is the con of low-fat products where the reality often belies the sales gimmick, as in yes, they will reduce the fat, but replace that fat with more sugar. If you try to find a processed product that is low in fat, salt and sugar, you will be looking until the twelfth of never; they don't exist you see. Cholesterol in the arteries is not just attributable to the heart. Poor diet and little exercise cause Small Vessel Disease (SVD) of the brain where signals malfunction because arteries in the brain are blocked, which in turn advances into memory deterioration and eventual dementia.

Decoding *The X Factor*

The current trend in media circles seems to be the debate around media literacy, which by one definition is the ability to effectively and efficiently comprehend and utilise mass media content. This includes an awareness of the impact of media, understanding the process of mass communication, understanding media content and being able to use strategies for analysing and discussing media messages.

For example, to relate it to today's tense, it is to make sense of, and even enjoy, media entertainment packages like ITV's *The X Factor*. It seems this show is not difficult to fathom. Regurgitated Ancient Roman themes where judge and jury (emperor-like figures that have the mere mortals' futures in their hands) presiding over a contest that the mob as the audience can overrule, is old-hat.

Am I media literate, one ponders: after all, I can see right through cheap spectacles like *The X Factor*? Even the audition stage has become predicable. People with apparently no self-respect warble any old thing; with some even aware how crass they are, but know that the baseness factor has an entertainment angle too, and some creepy old agent could be watching to make them a sort of ridiculed star.

Then we have the ones that make it through almost begging to get there. Oohing and ahhing at the judge's every word; because yes, they're all on a journey. And what the contestants would give to walk the same carpet as the A-listers; to gurgle in appreciation at that same A-lister making positive comments regarding their vocal capacities. And that contrived look of shock by the contestant should they win, to propagate to the masses (including those baying for blood) that they had not expected it; of course they must have at least half-expected to win or why did they enter?

Before that grand final may I add; the contesting wannabe must keep tight-lipped if they get a good barracking in case they get the standard thumbs down. After all, these 'celebrity' judges can secure them recording contracts – it's not what you know it's who you know. This can be seen with Louis Walsh and Simon Cowell. One contact I am glad I don't know is Simon Cowell's dentist; that strip of white marble for teeth is supposed to portray wealth. Hasn't your stylist told you yet, Simon, bright gapless veneers are so last Fall?

As for the acts themselves, well to be media literate in the televisual entertainment sense is to understand that you are nothing if you're not a star. The girl group, Hope (2008), seemed to sum it up in one. Initially a hotchpotch of rejects, perhaps they would have done better if they had gone one better and called themselves 'Desperadoes'. If they had they would have at least got one vote in my vote. Instead; to do the splits, whenever threatened with expulsion from the contest, brought a whole new literacy to understanding the entertainment industry.

Confronting her Fear

In Meek Mouse's village no one had ever been on holiday, let alone venture out to the other side of the county. All Meek Mouse had ever known was her wee hut in her wee familiar damp patch of the forest.

She wished that she had never won this damn vacation in the wheat-gathering contest. When she had entered the competition advocating wheat consumption defence she had no idea that she would win the darn thing.

Meek Mouse's little mouse-like teeth visibly chattered at the thought of her first flight out yonder. She could not eat that foreign grain was her justification for not venturing as far as the gatepost. But what could she do? After all, this socioeconomic environmental disaster occurring in her domain was all she knew.

The wheat was being deforested at an alarming rate.

She sighed as the visible barren landscape thundered around her ears from a mechanical contraption. Meek Mouse had to pretend not to notice the likeable rogue Leeching Lizard, and so she meekly meandered past, turning the other cheek.

"G'day," rasped Leeching Lizard in his broad Australian accent. "I hear you goin' abroad, whose flying yer, Eagle Star?"

Meek Mouse shook uncontrollably, then abruptly changed the subject and looked directly at Leeching Lizard.

"You look like you are half-starved, have you looked in the mirror lately?" said Meek Mouse.

Leeching Lizard's green cartilage bone audibly creaked as he strained his neck. Aghast became quite apparent in his large lizardy-like eyes.

"I know," he said.

Lizard then versed into mysterious narration as he collected his thoughts.

"Black smoke billowed like wild fire," he proceeded, "the Humans are razing the habitation, there's not a shoot to be seen, never mind a branch for me to leech, laze and scavenge on".

"It's looking bad."

"Anyway when you off?" he prompted.

"You're such a drama queen, Lizard," Meek Mouse chattered back. "I've never been abroad; they say bad things can happen during flight. Is it true, Lizard, you are a worldly sort?"

Lizard breathed into his hand and proudly rubbed his spindly breast bone.

"Nonsense," licked the lizard, lolling his tongue. "I told you months ago there was a holiday going for free called 'Wonderland'. It's free because all you do is dolly daydream about it. You can even take Tweedledum and Tweedledee along for the ride too. Anyway, the aircraft is fitted with stork-like stilts for rapid evacuation on impact, and a feather-fitted underbelly to water glide," added Lizard.

Meek Mouse moaned in helpless sarcastic anguish.

"That's made me feel heaps better."

"The meek shall inherit the earth," she had constantly reassured herself over the years.

Meek Mouse had to admit that she had admired Leeching Lizard for his brave adventures to dangerous boundaries afar. This unknown territory she was about to encounter because of this damn competition filled her with a nauseating dread.

Maybe it was only hearsay, but Meek Mouse did board her flight with Eagle Star. It was reported via the grapevine that she physically shook climbing the stairwell to board. Tentatively, as though walking the plank, she had tripped twice. Meek Mouse had sworn that she had spotted a flea in the wings of the craft but nobody had believed her; they said she was imagining things. The spread-eagled Eagle bade her to hold on tight and prepared the ascent. The craft on which Meek Mouse was travelling was fitted with the latest technology but did not make the jungle descent. Instead, a falling tree had felled the path and tending to a scratch had enabled collision. Meek Mouse had perished. The moral to this story is that Meek Mouse was duly right to be terrified of flight and should not have flown.

Confronting her terror had led to her demise.

Brogues, Monkey Boots, Tonics and the Panda Collar

I can remember the Top Rank days in Hanley, Stoke-on-Trent vividly; this dance club was open on Saturday mornings for children and open for children and early teens on a Tuesday night. I used to go in the years between 1972 and 1975, mostly on a Saturday morning.

To say it was the 'in' place to be would not do it justice. The odd time 'I got in' on a Tuesday night it was as though I had really come of age.

The popular groups around at this time were the Sweet, Slade and The Glitter Band and I was most definitely a Sweet fan (having experienced my musical epiphany with *Hell Raiser* in one of those little booths in Sherwin's music shop – now demolished). There were often competitions at Top Rank and I remember I entered one which featured the Sweet. One had to dress up like the characters in the group and I chose to dress like a Red Indian to illustrate *Wig Wam Bam*. The eventual winner, though, was a girl who had made one of those caped cloaks Steve Priest from the Sweet used to wear on stage. Yes, the winner was the contender who received the loudest cheer from the audience, made up of hundreds of children. Top Rank was always packed. Even under the stairs, where many a romance occurred in between the coats.

Your dress for the occasion had to be top rank and was of paramount importance in those days. The shop was Chawners on Hope Street, Hanley, where the clobber was not what one would call *vieux jeu*. The fashions of the day post-bellbottoms were parallels (the leg of the trouser was supposed to be parallel all the way down). There were also different names for the different colour trouser. We had Stones (a creamy colour), Wines, Petrol Blues, Bottle Greens and Canaries (yellow). There was also Tonics and Tonic Checks, Prince of Wales and Bakers (like a white jean). I also persuaded a friend to give me a 'feather cut' to match, which was the latest hairstyle of the time, but my mother was not a happy bunny on seeing the result and immediately sent me to the barbers to have it rectified.

I eventually opted for Wines (a maroon colour) and got a discount on my first pair because my cousin worked at the store. Ben Sherman shirts, as an accompaniment, were also fashionable in this epoch which sometimes sported the 'panda collar' (a massive flap-like shirt collar). Shoes-wise, it was Brogues and Monkey Boots to accompany your Harrington or Star jumper. Yes, life was sweet in the Top Rank days, your only worry being if you could enact your dance routine to the latest hits. These would include that caper where you put your hands on your hips and sort of rocked your arms as you bowed your head (I would never partake in this one; it was done by those Greaser or Frib types to tunes by Status Quo and the like). Then there was that dance to the Glitter Band where you moved your legs one behind the other in rhythm. The trendiest though, was to move one's feet slowly in a short forward step, then back again to the glam rock beat.

Those were the days; and I'm not referring to Mary Hopkin.

The Final Chapter

With regard to life, death and all that goes in between, I have always reasoned that maybe we have a succession of little lives, not one long one. When you cast your mind back to times gone by, it is as though we lived a different life in a different epoch. When one chapter ended, another one began. This can be seen when ending a relationship, moving location, getting a new job, giving up the booze or even redecorating.

Not many can determine when they are truly engaging with their final chapter. Furthermore, most of us have faith in some kind of God, with some even believing they will be born anew after death, by rebirth or reincarnation. Who wants to live by a secular or atheist doctrine in that we live and die and then we're done. Surely there must be more?

To close this manuscript, this, *The Final Chapter* article (hopefully not mine), was written in Kathmandu, Nepal. What better place to research rebirth and reincarnation? Even well-travelled ears tend to prick if one demonstrates cultural capital by declaring they are going to Kathmandu.

September 12th 2018 – Thamel, Kathmandu

I have little knowledge of the Buddhist or Hindu religions. Buddhism, in a sentence, advocates that suffering must endure, but one can transcend this pain with a spiritual awakening through meditation. Karma also figures highly for the Buddhists, as does rebirth, which is distinctively different from the Hindu idea of reincarnation.

Hedonic adaptation is also an interesting concept, which sits well with belief systems. Basically, hedonic adaptation means that the material objects we attain in life, we adapt to, so we then want more and more material objects to feel fulfilled. This can be exemplified by buying a terraced house, then we want a semi, then a detached, then a mansion, then two mansions. Materialism cannot fulfil – simple as.

As a forewarning, visitors to Kathmandu are not advised regarding the crippling natural earth (dust). On seeing many clearing their throats of phlegm (the onomatopoeia being 'archt tper') and then projecting spittle had me recoiling.

On my first morning in Kathmandu, I experienced not a spiritual awakening but an earthly one. My ongoing mild breathing difficulties brought out the hypochondriac in me, believing that perhaps I had the first symptoms of malaria (a strange insect welt was visible on my right ankle). After discussing it with reception staff at the hotel, it was found that the cause was the powdery fine earth. Usually scoffing at those wearing 'pollution masks' with the view that they were nothing more than exhibitionists, yours truly could be seen just one hour later emerging from the hotel also wearing a pollution mask. Now respecting the masked crusaders, I also had to enact the odd 'archt tper' to boot. This was about my health and I was taking no chances.

Turning back to the reincarnation theme: What's the use of coming back if you don't remember the last time around? I cannot remember being here before, can you? At any rate, are we being reborn through our children living on after our demise? In contrast, all family lines inevitably end when sooner or later, only one child will be conceived and through a range of factors will not reproduce, and as a result, the direct family line will cease to exist.

Going off piste a little, even if you are an only child, the trip over the sacrosanct Mount Everest for a one hour flight costing under £200 is a must do before you expire. Although I managed to snap the snap of all snaps over the highest peak in the world, the view of the Himalayas was slightly marred because of the cheap, discoloured windows of the aircraft. This was in stark contrast to the vista in the cockpit, of which we were invited in to take pictures. To advertise the mountain trip as 'Crystal Clear Views of Everest', complete with new window technology would generate even more interest in the event. It would cost, but one must speculate to accumulate. And no, I didn't put a complaint in.

There were no criticisms regarding the next trip. The temple excursion to visit the Buddhist Seto Machhendranath Temple and the Hindu Pashupatinath Temple on the banks of the Bagmati River was one of the most interesting days ever encountered. Firstly, one is immersed into the world of the Buddhist shrines at Seto, which include colour, sound, and strange aromas that had me questioning it all. Religion was fun, not authoritarian. There would then be another contradiction. Temple worshippers were throwing peelings and such in the direction of a terrified goat at a makeshift altar in readiness for sacrifice I was informed. The poor creature's troubled demeanour indicated it was well aware of its fate.

It would be the visit to the Hindu Pashupatinath Temple that would invite the biggest intrigue of all intrigues I would later discover. Looking on from the bridge and from the other side of the river with bemused amazement, as human bodies wrapped in orange (face showing) were being brought out and cremated on stone slabs by the Bagmati River, was a spectacle to beat all spectacles. A tour guide relayed that the funeral pyre is initially ignited from inside the deceased's mouth, and the cremation ritual is a purification process, in order that the now departed can be reincarnated. And to top it off, the ashes were then brushed into the river after the three-hour burning ceremony. The normalisation of the event added to the surreal naturality of it all. During the multiple cremations, onlookers ate banquets as monkeys and dogs sauntered by, all unconcerned by the mystical proceedings unfolding in their presence.

Yes, I had seen it all now. I know that being incinerated or buried are not exactly appealing inevitabilities to look forward to, but the riverside cremations seemed, well, so final.

The next port of call was a flight south to Chitwan National Park, which is situated in the buffer zone nearing the Indian border. Imagining Mowgli from The Jungle Book making an entrance at any time reinforced 'proper' jungle authenticity. The royal Bengal tiger, as well as rhinos and elephants, roamed the forests nearby.

During a worthy of note canoe trip, floating with the river current, I should not have had to point out to the tour guide that it was the sound of the jungle I had come to listen to, not noisy chatter from both the tour guides and tourists alike. I explained that I had already been exposed to a good dose of the crowds of human craziness in Kathmandu and it was not good for your health.

During a Jeep safari and discussing the monsoons, although abstract, it occurred that the natural elements (like the sun and the rain) were, perhaps, the real superior force in the great schematic scheme of things. Knowing where and when to shine and deluge, and to have sustained all life forms for millions of years is a miraculous accomplishment in itself, isn't it? Could we go as far as to say that the elements are also calculating, just like we believe our major deities do? Would we also dare to hazard that the natural elements are not just 'there' for us to harness and utilise, but are eternally assessing when to heat and when to water, with a view to regenerating and replenishing, at differing intervals. This would include reenergising all living organisms of all magnitudes, with the objective being to initiate new life cycles for all eternity. Is, therefore, natural ecological rejuvenation a form of rebirth or reincarnation?

Yes, there were challenging ideas and insights to grapple with in Nepal, including the animal question, which in my mind's eye, repeatedly reared its ugly head. Those devoutly believing that we are reincarnated as animals must be of the masochistic kind, considering the pain and suffering other animals endure in comparison to human beings. On learning that leopards came into the village to take sleeping domestic dogs off the streets as easy pickings (apparently, leopards are quite partial to dog), to see one chained elephant (at the Elephant Breeding Centre) behaving strangely with bizarre repetitive motions (going nuts) and bearing witness to buffalo and their young tied up in back yards or heading for the river for respite from swarms of tormenting flies, I would rather not come back if it's okay with you.

When discussing the elephant in leg irons with two (I think German) tourists, a little ruckus ensued. We all agreed (except the tour guide who made a valid point that we keep dogs on leashes) that we were not comfortable with the elephant's obvious distress. Regarding the wildlife safaris, I suggested that the animals could hear us coming (in the outmoded Jeeps) a mile away and would quickly disappear into the bush, which in turn, restricted our viewing chances. I suggested a rapid camouflaged cable car to travel quietly around the jungle to which the female of the two tourists laughed. I then asked if she would prefer the Jeep, to which she replied, "Oh no." Her argument was that we should not be going into the jungle to see the animals, period. I quickly retorted that most people want to engage with animals and if any long-term scheme regarding animal welfare was going to be successful it would have to be supported by the majority. We left it at that.

Later that evening, when dawdling by the Rapti River (famed for its spectacular sunsets) and reading the dos and don'ts regarding entry to Chitwan National Park got me thinking about trophy hunters and poachers who can be shot on site in Nepal. If 'stiff' shoot to kill penalties like this were introduced worldwide, what would the trophy hunter be subsequently reincarnated as, the appropriately named false clown beetle (this insect feeds on rotting corpses and excrement)? In this instance, the trophy hunter could gorge at leisure, not just on faeces, but on the now putrid carcass of the creature they had unnecessarily hunted down and slaughtered for fun or sport.

Now that would be appropriate reincarnatory karma.

Memoirs

In chronological order, my earliest recollections of literature were at a Stoke-on-Trent school in 1972 as a ten- or eleven-year-old, when as a whole class, we read *The Lion, the Witch and the Wardrobe* by C. S. Lewis out loud. I distinctly remember how exciting it was to find another fantasy world entrance via the back of a wardrobe. What also stood out for me was the character Edmund, who, being ten years old too, beguiled when seduced by Turkish Delight. I most likely accessed other books as a child, but it is about what stands out and remains in the long-term memory. At twelve or thirteen, I would obtain the Ladybird books, which included the *Sly Fox* and the *Little Red Hen*. Not to read myself (they were for a much younger age group) but to write my own ditties on the blank white space under the illustrations to make the stories more humorous. More seriously, at this juncture in my life, *William Peter Blatty on The Exorcist* was found interesting, more so because it was nicked from a bookshop on Rhyl's High Street. In later years it was discovered that this book was the actual screenplay of the most infamous horror movie of all time, but in effect, at the time, it was acquired for the illustrations and swear words it contained. In the year 1975, we would read out the coarse guttural swear word dialogue by the character Regan/Demon in a café for a laugh. In saying that, I was seriously interested in *The Exorcist* movie and could not wait to view it. During this epoch I would read often, opting for English novelists like James Herbert, who wrote *The Fog* and *The Rats*. For my part, stories that were set in England were more appealing, but I have to admit that I would skip read at times to quickly get to the whole point of the exercise – the erotic content.

Just before leaving school in 1978, I distinctly recall revising word for word *Under Milk Wood* by Dylan Thomas. It was revised line by line in order to regurgitate it for an exercise. The English teacher would later accuse me of cheating because the poem was replicated onto paper with 100% accuracy. It must be said that even though forced to undertake this exercise I cannot remember a single line of it today, so am not sure if the verse influenced me as a writer, being as by nature, I would reject such classic/highbrow material. Throughout my life, I have always had a taste for the gritty, realist working-class 60s and 70s drama such as *Kes* by Barry Hines. We in fact read *Kes* out loud in class at high school and consequently I processed the working-class storylines of the time by watching epics like *Boys from the Blackstuff* on TV.

In 1979, as an eighteen-year-old, I can remember reading Gore Vidal's *Caligula*, which was based on the film starring Malcolm McDowell. Primarily, it was for the most part read for the erotic depictions and uncensored, brutal Roman torture portrayals, which were quite fascinating.

Note: such was the page saturation of interesting material one hardly had to skip read. On a personal level, Caligula was not all about the sex and violence, the vernacular was appreciated. I also respected how the characters referred to one another both in the Senate and in the bedroom. 'My Lord,' 'Sire,' and other title references added to the book's appeal and influences me today when setting an English-speaking story in a foreign land. The Emperor Caligula's duplicitous relationship with Macro, Praetorian Prefect, also enthralled.

In my early-to mid-twenties I began to develop a board game and subsequently read the Oxford and military dictionaries to locate difficult words to add to the Manoeuvre Cards mechanism, which was designed to include a spelling test. Travel books like *Baedeker's Germany* were also studied, for me to be able to write a synopsis on my featured cities of the world included in my invention. This exercise was intense; with the travel synopses and spelling test later dropped from the game content altogether. It was not a completely wasted exercise, I might add; even now obscure and difficult words can be recalled, such as zeitgeist and semaphore, which have been utilised for articles. Local Victorian texts featuring puritan life in the Potteries in that era have also been of great interest. In saying that, there was and still is a paucity of such storylines featuring the lower classes, so newspaper articles and historical Internet pieces were researched online instead. During the late 1990s, I entered college and studied English language/literature, where I read and studied *King Lear* by William Shakespeare. I found Shakespeare elitist, uninspiring, overrated and much ado about nothing.

From college I enrolled at university as a mature student, where my academic vocabulary expanded quite a degree. Lecturers remarked how I had mastered the academic conventions with some distinction and I was even chosen as the most exceptional student in the whole of the university. Although by now a skip reader and extractor (extracting information from set texts for essay assignments) we would often study literature in class, where my intelligence became academically polished after acquainting myself with the writer/s under critical spotlight. It was learnt that the German scholars of the Frankfurt School of thought concentrated on social theory and philosophy, and I became adept at applying the School's theories to media and popular culture, which would inevitably encompass the Americanisation of British culture. What's more, arguments from Adorno and Marcuse regarding commodification, standardisation and false needs were applied to the videogame genre for my eventual MA dissertation, after extracting the relevant arguments espoused by the likes of Herbert Schiller in *Information Inequality: The Deepening Social Crisis in America* (1996).

Academic university prerequisites, stipulating that one must balance the argument when writing critically, became second nature, bearing in mind that there was the 'elitist' criticism of the school, in that Adorno was not as impoverished as the 'workers' he had notions on and could afford to engage in high cultural pastimes. One of my favourite authors on this subject was Dominic Strinati and his *An Introduction to Theories of Popular Culture*.

Although only reading short paragraphs, other authors reviewed while studying European Culture at university were Edgar Allan Poe and Franz Kafka. I managed to peruse *The Pit and the Pendulum* during a long-haul flight to the States and found it heavy going. The tale was set within the walls of a prison cell in Toledo, Spain, during the Spanish Inquisition. I understood where Poe was coming from and identified with his dark and morose mindset dictating his narrative, no doubt brought on by his numerous neurological disorders and substance abuse. To me he was most definitively a tortured soul. Contrastingly, Franz Kafka's *Metamorphosis* was explored in a European Culture module to some extent. Not getting Kafka at first, it would be years later that Kafka's hinted cynicism of humanity would be identified in *Metamorphosis*. I deduced that Kafka was sniping at the social order and the 'price of love' when describing how he was of no use to his demanding family once he was no longer the main breadwinner, having turned into a beetle.

At the turn of the 21st century, a taste for the factual accounts of Belfast journalist Martin Dillon was developed where all of Dillon's paperbacks, themed on the troubles in Northern Ireland, were scrutinised with some depth. Yes, I read the lot. This included *The Dirty War* and *The Trigger Men*, which detailed all the startling double standard peculiarities of war. To me Dillon's portrayals were a fascinating, enlightening reading experience where I became privy to the realities of this recent, bloody conflict enacted on our islands. It was a feeling of privilege uncovering the backdrop as to how double agents worked and the barbarous penalties meted out for those discovered. On the other hand, Dillon's journals could be a little unnerving, especially with regard to how innocent people were taken off the streets in West Belfast to be tortured and executed, as seen in *The Shankill Butchers*.

On another subject matter, my reading and writing life has always been interspersed with complaints (or bringing issues) to scores of institutions where I socially campaigned for greater accountability and transparency from representatives from housing, social care, disability, DWP, council, MPs, utility companies and high street stores. Now having the capability to take the representatives of these organisations to the wire, I would often attend high level appeals and tribunals where executives from the institution in question would attend.

Examining many of the replies from such institutions, then responding accordingly to their extenuation, centred my own style in being able to tackle the institutions effectively. One housing complaint, made because there had been voiced inappropriate comments from a housing officer, elicited a response stating: "In future the housing officer will be more circumspect with their phraseology." I found this turn of phrase very precise and was one of the few turn of phrases I would use myself (with slight variations) in later correspondence with other institutions.

Other than skip-reading responses to issues I had brought to notice (I don't like to use the word complaint because it has misleading connotations), I more or less stopped reading after attaining my MA in Media Futures in 2008. Post 2008, *The Damage Done* (1997) by Warren Fellows, in which an Australian drug smuggler endures the horrors of a Thai jail to tell the tale, was read and enjoyed. I also managed to reread it in 2016, which was an achievement in itself. The reason I enjoyed The Damage Done, is because the scene is set at the outset, where a French prisoner screeches in terror because a cockroach had burrowed into his ear to lay what was now a heaving lumped mass about to erupt from his neck. A true story, the barbarity repeatedly unfolded throughout the biography. Yes, I had been spoiled. An attempt to read a similar story, set in a Venezuelan jail, saw me abort after just a few pages because I did not have the time or the patience to read the idiosyncrasies to the build-up to the discovery of the drugs, like how one flies the mast on a yacht, for example.

Not only had my style by now been developed, there was not much more other authors could offer me. I had my own storylines.